Atlas of Diabetes Mellitus

This completely revised and updated fourth edition of the *Atlas of Diabetes Mellitus* provides broad coverage of all aspects of diabetes mellitus and an extensive collection of common and rare clinical images. It aims to provide an invaluable resource for anyone interested in the management of this ubiquitous clinical condition, including primary care/family physicians, endocrinologists, physicians in training, diabetic specialist nurses and other key professionals who are likely to be involved in the care of patients with diabetes mellitus.

Atlas of Diabetes Mellitus

Fourth Edition

Ian N. Scobie and David Hopkins

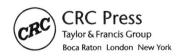

CRC Press
Taylor & Francis Group
Boca Raton London New York

CRC Press is an imprint of the
Taylor & Francis Group, an **informa** business

Cover images courtesy of Ian N Scobie and David Hopkins

Fourth edition published 2024
by CRC Press
2385 NW Executive Center Drive, Suite 320, Boca Raton FL 33431

and by CRC Press
4 Park Square, Milton Park, Abingdon, Oxon, OX14 4RN

CRC Press is an imprint of Taylor & Francis Group, LLC

© 2024 Ian N Scobie and David Hopkins

Third edition published by Informa Healthcare 2006

ISBN: 9781032379456 (hbk)
ISBN: 9781032379463 (pbk)
ISBN: 9781003342700 (ebk)

DOI: 10.1201/9781003342700

Contents

Author Biographies

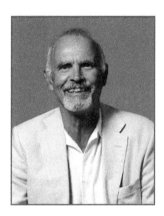

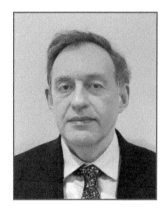

Dr Ian N. Scobie qualified MBChB and MD from the University of Glasgow, subsequently being elected a Fellow of the Royal College of Physicians of London. He trained in Internal Medicine and Endocrinology and Diabetes at the Glasgow Royal Infirmary and at St Thomas' Hospital, London. Dr Scobie was appointed as Consultant Physician in Medicine and Endocrinology and Diabetes at Medway Maritime Hospital, Kent, England, and later Honorary Senior Lecturer at King's College London School of Medicine related to his appointment as Clinical Sub-Dean responsible for undergraduate students at his institution. He also served as site director for The American University of the Caribbean School of Medicine between 2003 and 2009. Dr Scobie's research interest is in his specialty of endocrinology and diabetes, and he has published extensively in his field. He has authored and co-authored chapters in diabetes and metabolism and textbooks of diabetes. He has had a longstanding commitment to medical education at both the undergraduate and postgraduate level. Dr Scobie's current appointment is Assistant Clinical Dean, United Kingdom, American University of the Caribbean School of Medicine.

Dr David Hopkins is a consultant physician with more than 30 years of experience in clinical and academic diabetes. He qualified in medicine in Liverpool and completed specialty training in Liverpool and London. For most of his career, he has been associated with King's College London and its associated academic health science partnership, King's Health Partners, where he was a Director of the Institute of Diabetes, Endocrinology and Obesity from 2014 to 2022 and an Honorary Reader in Diabetic Medicine. He recently moved to Jersey, where he is leading the development of diabetes services for the island. He has held regional and national leadership positions in diabetes, notably as the medical chair of the Council of Healthcare Professionals at Diabetes UK from 2016 to 2023.

He has broad clinical and academic interests across the whole spectrum of diabetes, with particular focus on diabetes technology and psychosocial factors in diabetes care. He maintains close academic links with King's Health Partners and is diabetes lead for the Health Outcomes Observatory (H2O), an EU programme to develop a network of data observatories for long-term conditions across Europe.

Foreword

As a third-year medical student, I could not construe of a more boring disease than type 2 diabetes mellitus. After all, if this were merely a side-effect of sloth and gluttony, why expend effort in learning about it (and making it a part of one's career)? Further exposure to the disease and its complications disabused me of these impressions and also brought home the realization that a knowledge of diabetes would serve as a summary of most of internal medicine. With this in mind, it is certainly my pleasure to write the Foreword to the fourth edition of Dr Ian N. Scobie's *Atlas of Diabetes Mellitus*, co-authored by Dr David Hopkins. In doing so, I am following in the footsteps of my teacher, mentor and friend Dr Robert A. Rizza, to whom I owe the realization that diabetes is a complex, heterogenous disease with diverse contributions to its pathogenesis.

What is diabetes and why is it important? Let us answer the latter question first. Diabetes is well on its way to becoming, directly and indirectly, the most economically important chronic disease of the 21st century. Its contribution to the costs of care and the burdens of limb loss, blindness, renal failure and vascular disease are readily appreciated. Although the diagnosis is fairly straightforward, chronic therapy, coupled with the necessity to change behaviour, means that management can be anything but. In the past decade, progress has been made on multiple fronts in the treatment of this disease. However, the implementation of these advances is costly and complex, which means that they are far from becoming universal. Moreover, newer therapies may make subsets of the disease easier to treat but are far from curative—the

lessons imparted by the *Atlas of Diabetes Mellitus* remain very relevant.

What is diabetes? It is a unique disease defined by the presence of hyperglycaemia. Although, broadly speaking, there are two categories of diabetes—immune-mediated or type 1 diabetes and type 2 diabetes—it should be apparent that one is defined by the (imperfect) exclusion of the other. The complications of hyperglycaemia and hypoglycaemia are nevertheless common to both. Beyond overlap between type 1 and type 2 diabetes, there is significant heterogeneity in the causation of type 2 diabetes. While this may be obvious to the specialist, the generalist may not appreciate the subtle clues underlying a diagnosis of haemochromatosis- or acromegaly-associated diabetes. Similarly, specialists usually require years of experience to see and understand rare conditions, such as lipodystrophy, that are associated with diabetes. For these cases alone, *Atlas of Diabetes Mellitus* remains an invaluable contribution to the literature.

Although, or perhaps because, a picture is 'only' worth a thousand words, this book provides a depth and breadth to an overview of diabetes that will serve its readers well by facilitating the acquisition of new and useful information. Therefore, in conclusion, I would like to echo the Foreword of the previous edition where Dr. Rizza stated that '… those of you who choose to add this excellent Atlas to your library will find that you will also share my enthusiasm for this delightful book.'

Adrian Vella MD
Rochester, MN, US

Acknowledgments

Great thanks go to Professor Peter Sönksen and Dr Clara Lowy, formerly of St Thomas' Hospital, London, UK, who kindly supplied many of the images in this Atlas. Thanks also to Dr Tom Barrie, of The Glasgow Eye Infirmary, Glasgow, UK, who provided a splendid set of eye photographs (Chapter 8, Figures 8.2, 8.7, 8.18 and 8.20–8.22), Dr Alan Foulis, formerly of The Royal Infirmary in Glasgow, UK, who supplied some magnificent pathology images (Chapter 2, Figures 2.17–2.20, 2.23–2.27, 2.29–2.33, 2.35) and Eli Lilly and Company for providing a series of images (Chapter 1, Figures 1.1–1.3; Chapter 3, Figures 3.1–3.4 and 3.6–3.8).

We are grateful to the following who also contributed their images:

Professor Andrew Hattersley, University of Exeter Medical School, UK (Chapter 2, Figure 2.1), Dr Nick Finer, Luton and Dunstable Hospital, Bedfordshire, UK (Chapter 2, Figure 2.2); Professor Ian Campbell, Victoria Hospital, Kirkaldy, Fife, UK (Chapter 2, Figure 2.8 and Chapter 8, Figure 8.28); Dr Sam Chong, Medway Maritime Hospital, Gillingham, Kent, UK (Chapter 2, Figure 2.11); Drs Angus MacCuish and John Quin, formerly of The Royal Infirmary, Glasgow, UK (Chapter 2, Figure 2.12); Dr Julian Shield, University of Bristol, UK (Chapter 2, Figure 2.13); Professor Julia Polak, Royal Postgraduate Medical School, Hammersmith, London, UK (Chapter 2, Figures 2.21 and 2.22); Professor GianFranco Bottazzo, previously of The London Hospital Medical College, London, UK (Chapter 2, Figure 2.28); Dr Gray Smith-Laing (Chapter 2, Figures 2.36, 2.37 and 2.39) and Dr Richard Day, formerly of Medway Maritime Hospital, Gillingham, Kent, UK (Chapter 2, Figure 2.38); MiniMed, Ashtead, UK (Chapter 3, Figure 3.13); MediSense, Maidenhead, UK (Chapter 3, Figure 3.12); Dr David Kerr, Royal Bournemouth Hospital, Dorset, UK (Chapter 3, Figure 3.11); Professor Pratik Choudhary, University of Leicester (Chapter 3, Figure 3.20).

Dr William Campbell, Royal Victorian Eye & Ear Hospital, Melbourne, Australia (Chapter 8, Figures 8.10–8.12 and 8.16, 8.17); Professor Stephanie Amiel, King's College Hospital, London, UK (Chapter 6, Figure 6.4, Chapter 7, Figure 7.2, Chapter 10, Figure 10.1 and Chapter 12, Figures 12.1 and 12.2); Xeris Pharmaceuticals UK (Chapter 6, Figure 6.3a); Professor Peter Thomas, formerly of the Royal Free School of Medicine, Hampstead, London, UK (Chapter 8, Figure 8.25); Mr Grant Fullarton, Gartnavel General Hospital, Glasgow, UK (Chapter 8, Figure 8.32); Pfizer Limited, Sandwich, UK (Chapter 8, Figures 8.33–8.36); Dr Roger Lindley (Chapter 8, Figure 8.37); Dr Brian Ayres, formerly of St Thomas' Hospital, London, UK (Chapter 8, Figures 8.42 and 8.43); Dr Kumar Segaran, formerly of Medway Maritime Hospital, Gillingham, Kent, UK (Chapter 8, Figures 8.44 and 8.45); Mrs Ali Foster, formerly of King's College Hospital, London, UK (Chapter 8, Figure 8.46); Mr Mike Green (Chapter 8, Figures 8.47 and 8.48), Dr Kishore Reddy (Chapter 8, Figure 8.53), Dr Paul Ryan (Chapter 8, Figures 8.55 and 8.56), Dr Larry Shall (Chapter 8, Figures 8.58,

8.63–8.64, 8.66), all formerly of Medway Maritime Hospital, Gillingham, Kent, UK; Dr Peter Watkins, formerly of King's College Hospital, London, UK (Chapter 8, Figure 8.70); Mr Harry Belcher, Queen Victoria Hospital, East Grinstead, Sussex, UK (Chapter 8, Figure 8.72); Dr Annieke Van Barr Amsterdam University Medical Centre & Editorial team of *Gut* (Chapter 12, Figure 12.3); Dr Kelly White, Fractyl Health Inc, Lexington MA; (Chapter 12, Figure 12.4); Dr Bob Ryder, Sandwell & West Birmingham NHS Trust & GI Dynamics (Chapter 12, Figure 12.5).

Finally, thanks go to Mrs Daniella James, Mrs Carol Esson and Mrs Elizabeth Cannell for help with previous editions.

Dr Ian N. Scobie MD FRCP
Bearsted, Kent

Dr David Hopkins FRCP
Grouville, Jersey

Abbreviations

4S Trial	Scandinavian Simvastatin Survival Study	EDIC	Epidemiology of Diabetes Interventions and Complications study
ABBOS	Bovine serum albumin	EDKA	Euglycaemic diabetic ketoacidosis
AGP	Ambulatory glucose profile	ESRD	End-stage renal disease
ACC	American College of Cardiology	FDA	Food and Drug Administration
ACE	Angiotensin-converting enzyme	FFA	Free fatty acids
ACR	Albumin-to-creatinine ratio	FIELD	Fenofibrate Intervention and Event Lowering in Diabetes
ADA	American Diabetes Association		
AGEs	Advanced glycation end products	FINDIA	Finnish Dietary Intervention Trial for the Prevention of Type 2 Diabetes
ARB	Angiotensin receptor blocker		
BABY DIET	Primary Prevention of Type 1 Diabetes in Relatives at Increased Genetic Risk	FGF-19	Fibroblast growth factor 19
		FPG	Fasting plasma glucose
		GAD	Glutamic acid decarboxylase
BMI	Body mass index	GCK	Glucokinase
CAPD	Continuous ambulatory peritoneal dialysis	GDM	Gestational diabetes mellitus
		GIP	Gastrointestinal inhibitory polypeptide
CARDS	Collaborative Atorvastatin Diabetes Study		
		GLP-1	Glucagon-like peptide-1
CARE	Cholesterol and Recurrent Events Trial	GLUT4	Insulin-regulated glucose transporter
CHD	Coronary heart disease	GWAS	Genome-wide association studies
CKD	Chronic kidney disease	HHS	Hyperosmolar hyperglycaemic state
CTG	Cardiotocography	HLA	Human leucocyte antigen
CVD	Cardiovascular disease	HMG-CoA	Hydroxymethylglutaryl-coenzyme A
DAFNE	Dose adjustment for normal eating	HNF	Hepatocyte nuclear factor
DAISY	Diabetes Autoimmunity Study in the Young	HNS	Hyperglycaemic hyperosmolar nonketotic syndrome
DCCT	Diabetes Control and Complications Trial	HONK	Hyperglycaemic hyperosmolar nonketotic coma
DESMOND	Diabetes Education and Self-Management for Ongoing & Newly Diagnosed diabetes	HPS	Heart Protection Study
		IA-2	Antibodies to tyrosyl phosphatase
		IAA	Insulin autoantibodies
DKA	Diabetic ketoacidosis	IAAP	Islet amyloid polypeptides
DM	Diabetes mellitus	IAK	Islet after kidney transplantation
DMR	Duodenal mucosal resurfacing	ICA	Islet cell antibodies
DVLA	Driver and Vehicle Licencing Agency	IDDM	Insulin-dependent diabetes mellitus
EASD	European Association for the Study of Diabetes	IDL	Intermediate-density lipoprotein
		IFG	Impaired fasting glucose
ED	Erectile dysfunction	IFN	Interferon

IGT	Impaired glucose tolerance	PCSK9	Proprotein convertase subtilisin/kexin type 9
IL	Interleukin		
INS	Proinsulin gene	PDE	Phosphodiesterase
KATP	ATP-sensitive potassium channel	PNDM	Permanent prenatal diabetes mellitus
LADA	Latent autoimmune diabetes of adulthood	RAAS	Renin-angiotensin-aldosterone system
LMWH	Low molecular weight heparin	RNA	Ribonucleic acid
Lp(a)	Lipoprotein A	SBP	Systolic blood pressure
MHC	Major histocompatibility complex	SPK	Simultaneous pancreas and kidney transplantation
MI	Myocardial infarction		
MODY	Maturity-onset diabetes of the young	SGLT	Sodium-glucose co-transporter
MRI	Magnetic resonance imaging	T1DM	Type 1 diabetes mellitus
MRSA	Methicillin-resistant *Staphylococcus aureus*	T2DM	Type 2 diabetes mellitus
		TCC	Total contact cast
NADiA	National diabetes inpatient audit	TNDM	Transient neonatal diabetes mellitus
NAFLD	Non-alcoholic fatty liver disease	TNF	Tumour necrosis factor
NASH	Non-alcoholic steatohepatosis	TRIGR	Trial to Reduce IDDM in the Genetically at Risk
NDM	Neonatal diabetes mellitus		
NIDDM	Non-insulin-dependent diabetes mellitus	UKPDS	United Kingdom Prospective Diabetes Study
NIP	Nutritional intervention to prevent	VEGF	Vascular endothelial growth factor
NSAID	Non-steroidal anti-inflammatory drug	VLDL	Very-low-density lipoprotein
OGTT	Oral glucose tolerance test	WHO	World Health Organisation
PAID scale	Problem Areas in Diabetes scale	ZnT8	Antibodies to zinc transporter

1

Introduction

Diabetes mellitus (DM) is recognised as one of the world's biggest health issues with immense social and economic consequences owing to the ever-increasing burden of new cases. The year 2022 saw the 100th anniversary of the discovery of insulin in Toronto, Canada. In the ensuing century, great progress has been made in the understanding of this ubiquitous condition, but still there remains no cure for type 1 diabetes mellitus (T1DM) and scant hope for most people with type 2 diabetes mellitus (T2DM) being able to reverse their condition (Figures 1.1–1.3).

The word *diabetes* means 'to run through' or 'a siphon' in Greek, and the condition has been recognised since the time of the ancient Egyptians. *Mellitus* (from the Latin and Greek roots for 'honey') was later added to the name of this disorder when it became appreciated that diabetic urine tasted sweet.

An epidemic of T2DM has occurred throughout the world, particularly affecting developing countries and migrants from these countries to industrialised societies. T2DM is more prevalent in people of lower socioeconomic status, and its prevalence

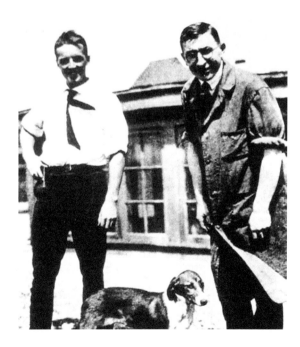

Figure 1.1 The discovery of insulin in 1922 is accredited to Frederick Banting (above right) and Charles Best (a medical student, above, left), supervised by JJR MacLeod and assisted by James Collip. The work was carried out at the University of Toronto.

DOI: 10.1201/9781003342700-1

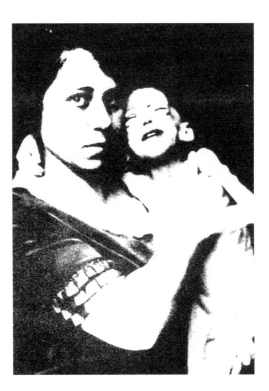

Figure 1.2 A 3-year-old child with type 1 diabetes mellitus, photographed in 1922 before insulin treatment was available. The only treatment then was a 'starvation' diet; patients rarely survived for more than 2 years.

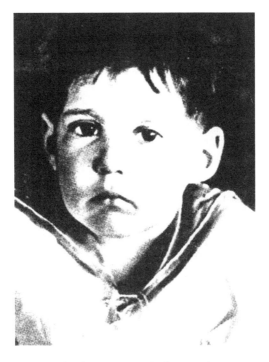

Figure 1.3 The same child as seen in the figure in 1923 after insulin treatment became available following its discovery by the Toronto group. The effect of this new therapy was 'miraculous'.

is rising more rapidly in low- and middle-income countries. Among the US population, crude estimates for the prevalence of diabetes for 2019 estimate that 8.7% of the population has diabetes. The prevalence is highest among American Indians and Alaska Natives (14.5%), followed by non-Hispanic Blacks (12.1%), people of Hispanic origin (11.8%), non-Hispanic Asians (9.5%) and non-Hispanic Whites (7.4%). According to a population-based study, 0.5% of US adults had diagnosed T1DM while 8.5% had diagnosed T2DM. As of 2019, the prevalence of diabetes in the UK was 7% of the population, but it will have risen since.

The incidence of T1DM differs enormously between populations. The world incidence rate is estimated at 15 per 100,000 people with particularly high incidence rates in Finland, Sweden and Saudi Arabia. There is a male preponderance (male to female ratio 1.8:1). There are peaks of incidence before school age and around puberty, with the diagnosis being made more frequently in spring and winter months. Modelling data in US children aged less than 20 years showed that the overall incidence of T1DM for the period 2002–2015 significantly increased as did, perhaps more alarmingly, T2DM.

The personal costs and costs to society of diabetes are very high. Out of every $4 in US health costs, $1 is spent caring for people with diabetes. Each year, $237 billion is spent on direct medical costs and $90 billion on reduced productivity. The UK, with its smaller population, spends £10 billion on diabetes care, around 10% of the annual National Health Service budget.

DEFINITION OF DIABETES

DM is a group of metabolic disorders characterised by hyperglycaemia. The hyperglycaemia results from defects in insulin secretion, insulin action or both. The chronic hyperglycaemia of diabetes is associated with specific chronic complications, resulting in damage to or failure of various organs, notably the eyes, kidneys, nerves, heart and blood vessels.

DIAGNOSIS OF DIABETES

The diagnostic criteria for DM were confirmed by the American Diabetes Association (ADA) in 2021. In clinical practice, establishing the diagnosis of diabetes is seldom a problem. When symptoms of hyperglycaemia exist (thirst, polyuria, weight loss, etc.), a random plasma glucose concentration of ≥11.1 mmol/l (200 mg/dl) or a fasting plasma glucose (FPG) of ≥7.0 mmol/l (126 mg/dl) confirms the diagnosis. Where diagnostic difficulty exists, the precise diagnosis can be established with an oral glucose tolerance test (OGTT) using a 75 g anhydrous glucose load dissolved in water: a 2-hour value ≥11.1 mmol/l (200 mg/dl) establishes the diagnosis of diabetes. An alternative criterion for the diagnosis of diabetes is a HbA_{1C} of 48 mmol/l ($\geq6.5\%$) using a measurement method that is certified by the NGSP (https://ngsp.org/) and standardised to the Diabetes Control and Complications Trial (DCCT) assay. Ideally, a confirmatory test using one of the other methods should be employed. The OGTT is not recommended for routine clinical use but may be an important test for epidemiological purposes where using only the FPG may lead to lower prevalence rates than with the combined use of the FPG and OGTT.

Prediabetes is a term used to denote individuals whose glucose levels do not meet the criteria for diabetes but are too high to be considered normal. Patients with prediabetes may fall into three categories. They may exhibit impaired fasting glucose (IFG) defined as a fasting plasma glucose between 5.6 mmol (100 mg/dl) and 6.9 mmol/l (125 mg/dl) or they may have a plasma glucose of 7.8 mmol/l (140 mg/dl) to 11.0 mmol/l (199 mg/dl) at 2 hours during a 75 g OGTT (impaired glucose tolerance or IGT). A further category includes those individuals who have a random HbA_{1C} of 39–47 mmol/l (5.7–6.4%). It is important to state that prediabetes is not to be considered a clinical entity or diagnosis, but rather a set of criteria conferring an increased risk of future diabetes and cardiovascular disease (Figure 1.4).

CLASSIFICATION OF DIABETES

The diagnostic label DM refers not to a unique disease, but rather to multiple disorders of different causation. Increasing knowledge has allowed us to identify discrete conditions caused by specific genetic abnormalities, while other types of diabetes remain difficult to classify on an aetiological basis. The ADA has published an aetiological classification of diabetes, an adapted version of which is presented in Figure 1.5.

Diagnosis of diabetes mellitus positive if:

Symptoms of diabetes plus random plasma glucose concentration of ≥11.1 mmol/l

or

Fasting plasma glucose concentration of ≥7.0 mmol/l

or

Plasma glucose concentration at 2 h ≥11.1 mmol/l during a 75 g oral glucose tolerance test
(in the absence of unequivocal hyperglycaemia or symptoms, the diagnosis should be
confirmed by repeat testing on a different day)

Figure 1.4 Although a definitive diagnosis of diabetes may be made using the glucose tolerance test, it is no longer recommended for routine clinical use. In the presence of diabetic symptoms, the diagnosis may be established by finding a random plasma glucose level of ≥11.1 mmol/l (200 mg/dl) or a fasting plasma glucose level of ≥7.0 mmol/l (126 mg/dl). Both impaired fasting glucose and impaired glucose tolerance are defined in the text.

T1DM (previously insulin-dependent diabetes mellitus [IDDM]) is characterised by autoimmune β-cell destruction, usually leading to absolute insulin deficiency and associated with a usually juvenile onset, a tendency to ketosis and diabetic ketoacidosis and an absolute need for insulin treatment. Most patients have type 1A diabetes, which is caused by a cellular-mediated autoimmune destruction of the β-cells of the pancreas and a minority have type 1B diabetes, the precise aetiology of which is not known. Latent Autoimmune Diabetes of Adulthood (LADA) is a form of T1DM which may initially be confused with T2DM (discussed below).

T2DM (previously non-insulin-dependent diabetes mellitus [NIDDM]) is associated with obesity and an onset later in life (although cases in childhood are now being recognised in the US and elsewhere). Patients, at least initially and often throughout their lives, do not have a need for insulin therapy to preserve life. The disorder is due to a progressive loss of adequate β-cell insulin secretion frequently on a background of insulin resistance. A precise cause (or causes) has not been found. This type of diabetes frequently remains undiagnosed for many years despite affected individuals being at risk of developing serious macrovascular or microvascular complications of the disease. Some patients may masquerade as T2DM patients, but ultimately are recognised as having a late-onset slowly progressing immune-mediated T1DM, so called latent

autoimmune diabetes of adulthood or latent autoimmune diabetes in adults (LADA).

Specific monogenetic defects of the β-cell have been identified and usually give rise to maturity-onset diabetes of the young (MODY). MODY is defined as a genetic defect in β-cell function subclassified according to the specific gene involved and is described in detail in Chapter 2.

Diabetes may result from any process that adversely affects the pancreas and such acquired processes include pancreatitis, trauma, pancreatectomy and pancreatic cancer. Usually, extensive pancreatic damage or removal must occur for diabetes to emerge. Cystic fibrosis, haemochromatosis and fibrocalculous pancreatopathy may also cause diabetes. Diabetes may also be caused by other endocrine diseases, particularly when there is over-secretion of hormones that antagonise the normal effect of insulin (including Cushing's syndrome, acromegaly, phaeochromocytoma). Drugs that have a similar effect (glucocorticoids, diazoxide, thiazides) or chemicals may also cause diabetes. Diabetes may also occur as a result of certain rare disorders associated with abnormalities of insulin or the insulin receptor, causing extreme insulin resistance and are sometimes found in association with acanthosis nigricans. These disorders are categorised as insulin resistance syndromes. There is a wide array of other genetic syndromes sometimes associated with diabetes, e.g. Down's, Klinefelter's and Turner's syndromes.

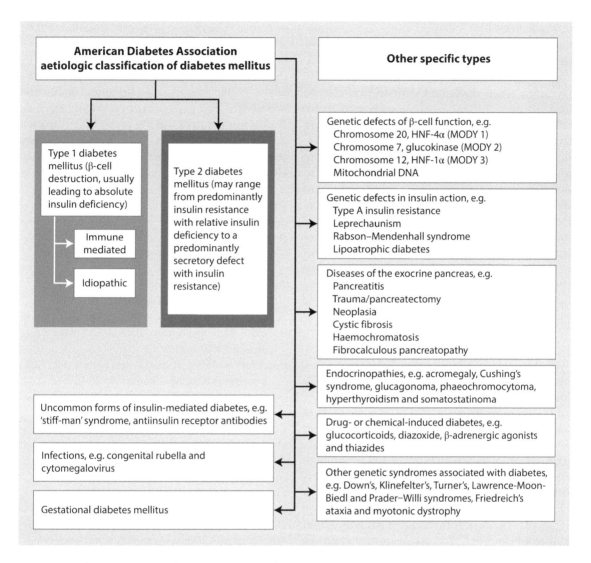

Figure 1.5 The American Diabetes Association has proposed an aetiological classification of diabetes based on research findings over the past two decades. The nomenclature has changed from insulin-dependent diabetes to type 1 diabetes and from non-insulin diabetes mellitus to type 2 diabetes. All forms of diabetes are characterised according to their known aetiologies, immunologic, genetic or otherwise. This opens up the concept of 'the diabetic syndrome'. HNF, hepatic nuclear factor; MODY, maturity-onset diabetes of the young.

Gestational diabetes mellitus (GDM) is normally defined as any degree of glucose intolerance with onset or first recognition during pregnancy. However, recent evidence suggests that many cases of GDM are in individuals with preexisting hyperglycaemia detected by routine screening in pregnancy and perhaps related to the prevalence of obesity. Care must be taken to exclude T2DM that was present before pregnancy and T1DM diagnosed during pregnancy. The patient's glucose tolerance status needs to be re-classified 6 weeks after giving birth. Deterioration of glucose tolerance occurs during normal pregnancy, especially in the third trimester. The criteria for diagnosing abnormal glucose tolerance in pregnancy have not been universally agreed upon worldwide: in the US, the modified O'Sullivan–Mahan criteria have been adopted, but these are at variance with the World Health Organization criteria. Patients with GDM are at future risk of developing T2DM.

Prediabetes (not a clinical entity but comprising IFG and IGT) refers to a pathophysiological state between normality and frank diabetes. Patients with IGT may only manifest as hyperglycaemic when challenged with an oral glucose load. Between 5–10% of people with prediabetes will progress to frank diabetes annually, although conversion rates vary by population characteristics. Although some may return to normal glucose tolerance, it is thought that most will be likely to develop diabetes eventually without significant lifestyle changes. Patients with IGT do not normally develop the microvascular complications of diabetes. However, they commonly display other features of the insulin resistance syndrome (also known as syndrome X, the metabolic syndrome or Reaven's syndrome), e.g. hypertension and dyslipidaemia, and IGT is associated with a major increase in cardiovascular risk.

EPIDEMIOLOGY OF DIABETES

The epidemiology of T1DM is complex. The overall incidence rates are comparable in North America and Europe; however, this disguises some marked variations in incidence rates between countries and even within countries. Within Europe, particularly high incidence rates are found in Finland, Sweden and Sardinia. Most Asian populations have a low incidence rate. In general, the incidence of T1DM seems to be increasing with an average increase in incidence of around 3% per year. About half of all cases of T1DM are diagnosed at an age of <15 years, with an observed peak in incidence rates in children aged 10–14 years. More recently, many cases are being diagnosed in children of <5 years of age. In many high-risk populations a male excess of T1DM is seen, especially after the age of puberty.

Cases of T2DM greatly exceed those of T1DM, accounting for about 85% of cases in Europe and significantly more in certain ethnic groups. It is estimated that 415 million people are living with diabetes worldwide, and this is projected to increase to half a billion by 2040, with a preponderance of cases in the developing world. In many populations, there is a declining age of peak incidence with cases now being identified in children and young adolescents, especially in highly susceptible groups such as Native Americans. In North America, T2DM is highly prevalent in Native American communities such as the Pima Indians, a feature shared by the Nauru and Papua New Guinea populations of the Pacific Islands. US Hispanics, Blacks and Polynesians also exhibit high prevalence rates. In 2019, it was reported that 7% of the UK population was living with diabetes. Higher rates have been observed in the South Asian population as reported also in the Indian subcontinent.

BIBLIOGRAPHY

American Diabetes Association. Type 2 diabetes in children and adolescents. Diabetes Care. 2000; 23: 381–9

American Diabetes Association. Classification and diagnosis of diabetes: standards of medical care in diabetes-2021. Diabetes Care. 2021; 44 (Supplement_1): S15–S33 https://doi.org/10.2337/dc21-S002

Bao W. Prevalence of diagnosed type 1 and type 2 diabetes among US adults in 2016 and 2017: population based study. BMJ. 2018; 362. doi: https://doi.org/10.1136/bmj.k1497

Centers for Disease Control and Prevention. National Diabetes Statistics Report. https://www.cdc.gov/diabetes/data/statistics-report/index.html

Eisenbarth GS. Type I diabetes mellitus. A chronic autoimmune disease. N Engl J Med. 1986; 314: 1360–8

MacFarlane IA. Diabetes mellitus and endocrine disease. In Pickup J, Williams G, eds. Textbook of Diabetes. Oxford: Blackwell Scientific Publications, 1991: 263–75

Mobasseri M, Shirmohammad M, Amiri T et al. Prevalence and incidence of type 1 diabetes in the world: a systematic review and meta-analysis. 10.34172/hpp.2020.18

Whicher CA, O'Neill SO, Holt RIG. Diabetes in the UK: 2019. Diabet Med. 2020 Feb; 37(2): 242–247. doi: 10.1111/dme.14225

Zimmet PZ, Tuomi T, Mackay IR, et al. Latent autoimmune diabetes mellitus in adults (LADA): The role of antibodies to glutamic acid decarboxylase in diagnosis and prediction of insulin dependency. Diabet Med. 1994; 11: 299–303

2

Pathogenesis

TYPE 1 DIABETES MELLITUS

Type 1 diabetes mellitus (T1DM) is a disorder of multifactorial causation: genetic, environmental and immunological. Worldwide, there is a marked geographical variation in prevalence. The overall prevalence in the general population is 0.4%. T1DM is caused by an interaction between environmental factors, an inherited genetic predisposition and unknown factors resulting in autoimmune destruction of the beta (β) cells of the endocrine pancreas (Figure 2.1).

Genetic factors

Only 10–15% of patients have a first- or second-degree relative with T1DM, so most patients do not have a family history of T1DM. In monozygotic

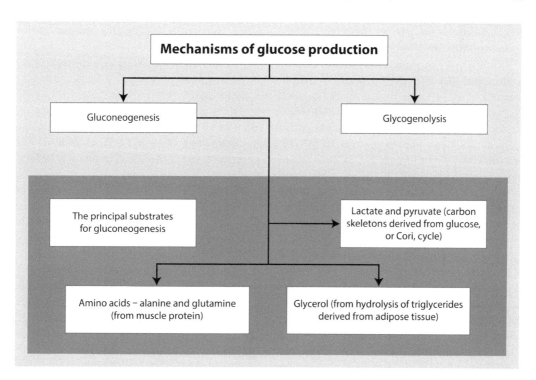

Figure 2.1 Glucose is produced in the liver by the process of gluconeogenesis and glycogenolysis. The main substrates for gluconeogenesis are the glucogenic amino acids (alanine and glutamine), glycerol, lactate and pyruvate. Many factors influence the rate of gluconeogenesis; it is suppressed by insulin and stimulated by the sympathetic nervous system. Glycogenolysis (the breakdown of hepatic glycogen to release glucose) is stimulated by glucagon and catecholamines, but is inhibited by insulin.

DOI: 10.1201/9781003342700-2

twins, the lifetime risk of developing T1DM is about 50%, the high discordance rate suggesting that other risk factors are at play. The risk to a first-degree relative is approximately 5–6%. Environmental triggers may account for up to two-thirds of the disease susceptibility.

In genome-wide association studies (GWAS) and meta-analyses, more than 50 T1DM genetic risk loci were identified. The strongest reported linkages for T1DM are within the major histocompatibility complex (MHC) region also known as human leucocyte antigen (HLA) located on chromosome 6. HLA complex polymorphic alleles are responsible for 40–50% of the genetic risk of the development of T1DM. Other genes are responsible for another 15% of the genetic predisposition, including the insulin gene (Ins-VNTR, IDDM2) polymorphisms on chromosome 11 and the cytotoxic T lymphocyte-associated antigen-4 gene (CTLA-4) on chromosome 2.

More than 90% of patients who develop T1DM have either HLA-DR3, DQB1*0201 (DR3-DQ2) or HLA-DR4, DQB1*0302 (DR4-DQ8) haplotypes, whereas fewer than 40% of normal controls have these haplotypes. DR3/DR4 heterozygosity is highest in children who develop diabetes before the age of 5 years (50%) and lowest in adults presenting with T1DM (20–30%) compared with an overall US population prevalence of 2.4%. Specific polymorphisms of the *DQB1* gene encoding the β-chain of class II DQ molecules predispose to diabetes in Caucasians but not in Japanese. In contrast, other DR4 alleles, such as DRB1*0403 and DPB1*0402 reduce the risk of developing T1DM even in the presence of the DQB1*0302 high-risk allele. HLA antigens (classes I and II) are cell-surface glycoproteins that play a crucial role in presenting autoantigen peptide fragments to T lymphocytes, thus initiating an immune response. Polymorphisms in the genes encoding specific peptide chains of the HLA molecules may therefore modulate the ability of β-cell-derived antigens to trigger an autoimmune response against the β-cell.

Polymorphisms located on the short arm of chromosome 11 close to the gene encoding for proinsulin may account for about 10% of the genetic predisposition of T1DM. This polymorphic site comprises a variable number of tandem repeats (Insulin-VNTR). Another gene, CTLA-4 (cytotoxic T lymphocyte antigen-4), located on the short arm of chromosome 2 (2q33), is also associated with the risk of developing T1DM. Other genetic associations include PTPN22, FoxP3, AIRE (autoimmune regulator, mainly expressed in the thymus marrow), STAT3, HIP14, ERBB3 and IFIH1.

Environmental factors

Strong evidence for the role of environmental factors in the causation of T1DM comes from the fact that the occurrence of T1DM in siblings who are monozygotic twins is around 50%. It remains unclear what the precise mode of action is for environmental factors. The most likely environmental factor implicated in the causation of T1DM is viral infection. It is noteworthy that children exposed to rubella in fetal life have an increased incidence of T1DM. RNA or proteins from viruses have been detected in the pancreas of patients with T1DM. Numerous viruses attack the pancreatic β-cell either directly through a cytolytic effect or by triggering an autoimmune attack against the β-cell. Evidence for a viral factor in aetiology has come from animal models and, in humans, from observation of seasonal and geographical variations in the onset of the disease. In addition, patients newly presenting with T1DM may exhibit serological evidence of viral infection. Viruses that have been linked to human T1DM include mumps, coxsackie B, retroviruses, rubella, cytomegalovirus and Epstein–Barr virus (Figures 2.2 and 2.3).

The 17-amino acid peptide ABBOS (bovine serum albumin), a major constituent of cow's milk, has been implicated as a cause of T1DM in children exposed at an early age, but definitive proof is lacking and this remains controversial. Nitrosamines (found in smoked and cured meats) and nitrate exposure from water intake may be diabetogenic as may chemicals known to be toxic to pancreatic β-cells, including alloxan, streptozotocin and the rat poison Vacor. Other environmental factors implicated in the development of T1DM include early ingestion of cereal or gluten in the diet, inadequate intake of omega-3 fatty acids and vitamin D deficiency (although vitamin D supplementation does not confer protection). Differences in the gut microbiota may also be involved in the pathogenesis of T1DM.

T1DM is associated with autoimmune destruction of the β-cells of the endocrine pancreas, most probably via apoptosis. Examination of islet tissue obtained from pancreatic biopsy or at postmortem from patients with recent-onset T1DM confirms a mononuclear cell infiltrate (termed insulitis) with

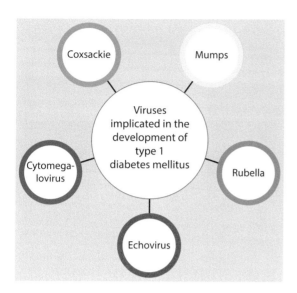

Figure 2.2 Viruses have been suggested to be a cause or factor in the development of type 1 diabetes mellitus (T1DM) and are thought to be the most likely agents to trigger the disease, probably on the basis of genetic predisposition, in some cases. Evidence comes from epidemiological studies and the isolation of viruses from the pancreas of a few recently diagnosed T1DM patients. Mumps and coxsackie viruses can cause acute pancreatitis, and coxsackievirus can cause β-cell destruction.

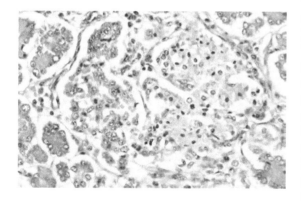

Figure 2.3 Autopsy sample of histology of coxsackie B viral pancreatitis in a neonate. Coxsackie B viral infection may cause inflammatory destruction of the β-cells and coxsackie B viruses have been isolated from the pancreas of patients with new-onset type 1 diabetes mellitus (T1DM). Injection of such isolates into mice causes insulitis and β-cell damage. Nevertheless, although coxsackie B virus may be diabetogenic in men, its precise aetiological importance in the development of T1DM remains unclear.

the presence of CD4 and CD8 T lymphocytes, B lymphocytes and macrophages, suggesting that these cells have a role in the destruction of β-cells. This chronic atrophic inflammation within the islets of Langerhans evolves over months or years while the patient remains euglycaemic, hyperglycaemia diagnostic of T1DM only emerging after a long latency period, reflecting the large number of β-cells that need to be destroyed before symptomatic diabetes ensues. Although the precise mechanism of such an insult has not been elucidated, it seems likely that an environmental factor, such as a viral infection, in a subject with an inherited predisposition to the disease, triggers the damaging immune response whereby β-cell components are recognised as autoantigens. This results in aberrant expression of class 1 and 11 major histocompatibility complexes (MHC) antigen by pancreatic β-cells. T lymphocytes recognise antigen-presenting cells and are activated, producing proinflammatory cytokines such as interleukin (IL)-2, interferon (IFN)γ and tumour necrosis factor (TNF)-α. (Other cytokines may be involved such as IL-6, IL-17 and IL-21, while others may confer protection.) A clone of T lymphocytes is generated that carries receptors specific to the presented antigen. Such T-helper cells assist B lymphocytes to produce antibodies directed against the β-cell. Such antibodies include islet cell antibodies (ICA) directed against cytoplasmic components of the islet cells. ICA presence may precede the development of T1DM. Some subjects may develop ICA temporarily and not go on to develop the disease, but persistence of ICA leads to progressive β-cell destruction associated with insulitis. T1DM ensues. Other antibodies associated with T1DM are islet cell-surface antibodies, insulin autoantibodies (IAA) and antibodies to an isoform of glutamic acid decarboxylase (GAD), found in approximately 70% of patients with autoantibody positivity at the time of diagnosis, antibodies to tyrosyl phosphatase (IA-2), found in approximately 60%, and antibodies to zinc transporter (ZnT8), found in 60–80% of newly presenting patients. In an analysis of data from three prospective cohort studies, 84% of children with two or more islet autoantibodies developed diabetes over 15 years of follow-up, hence the presence prior to diagnosis of two or three autoantibodies confers a greatly increased risk of progressing to T1DM. Screening children for T1DM has been suggested as a possible strategy with the added benefit

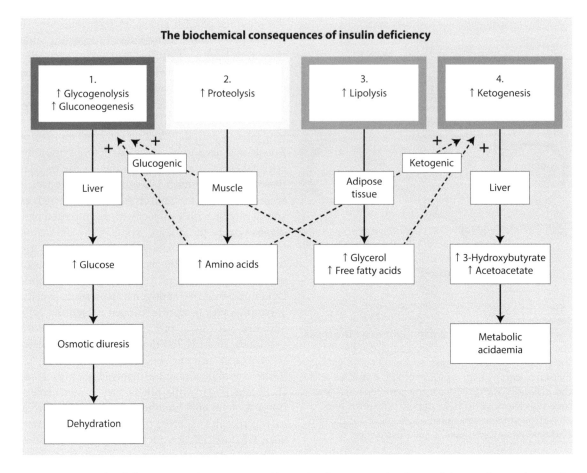

The biochemical consequences of insulin deficiency

| 1. ↑ Glycogenolysis ↑ Gluconeogenesis | 2. ↑ Proteolysis | 3. ↑ Lipolysis | 4. ↑ Ketogenesis |

Figure 2.4 Insulin deficiency results in increased hepatic glucose production and, hence, hyperglycaemia by increased gluconeogenesis and glycogenolysis. Insulin deficiency also results in increased proteolysis releasing both glucogenic and ketogenic amino acids. Lipolysis is increased, elevating both glycerol and non-esterified fatty acid levels which further contribute to gluconeogenesis and ketogenesis, respectively. The end result is hyperglycaemia, dehydration, breakdown of body fat and protein, and acidaemia.

of preventing children presenting with diabetic ketoacidosis which has been associated with worse glycaemic outcomes long term (Figures 2.4–2.17).

TYPE 2 DIABETES MELLITUS

Although genetic predisposition plays a role in the development of type 2 diabetes mellitus (T2DM), the main risk factors are obesity, low physical activity and an unhealthy diet. Several T2DM GWAS have clearly demonstrated the complex polygenic nature of T2DM in which most of the loci increase T2DM risk through reducing insulin secretion while a minority act through reducing insulin action. No genome-wide scans have identified any region with an effect as large as the HLA region in T1DM, so the exact mode of inheritance remains to be elucidated.

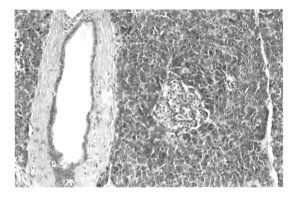

Figure 2.5 Constituents of a normal pancreas, medium-power view: to the left lies an excretory duct and, to the right, there is an islet surrounded by exocrine acinar cells. Haematoxylin and eosin stain.

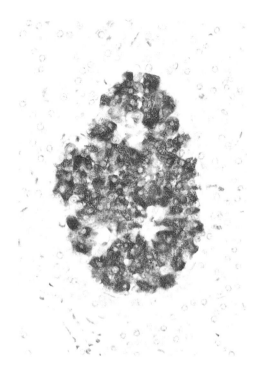

Figure 2.6 Normal islet immunostained for insulin. The majority (80%) of the endocrine cells are β-cells.

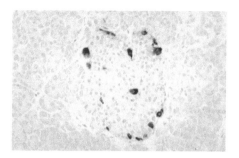

Figure 2.8 Normal islet immunostained for somatostatin. Somatostatin is contained in the D cells which are scattered within the islet. Somatostatin has an extremely wide range of actions. It inhibits the secretion of insulin, growth hormone and glucagon and also suppresses the release of various gut peptides. Somatostatinomas (D cell tumours) cause weight loss, malabsorption, gallstones, hypochlorhydria and diabetes.

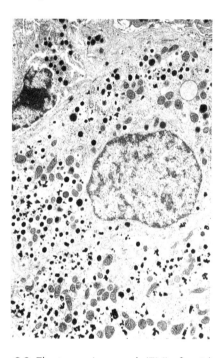

Figure 2.9 Electron micrograph (EM) of an islet of Langerhans from a normal pancreas showing mainly insulin storage granules in a pancreatic β-cell. A larger α-cell is also seen. The normal adult pancreas contains around 1 million islets comprising mainly β-cells (producing insulin), α-cells (glucagon), D cells (somatostatin) and pancreatic polypeptide (PP) cells. Islet cell types can be distinguished by various histologic stains and by the EM appearances of the secretory granules (as seen here). They can also be identified by immunocytochemical staining of the peptide hormones on light or electron microscopy (see Figures 2.12 and 2.13).

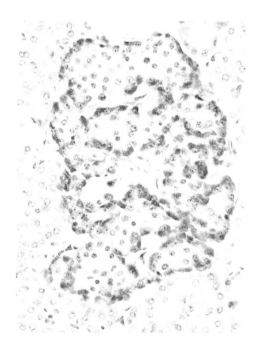

Figure 2.7 Normal islet immunostained for glucagon. Note that the α-cells mark the periphery of blocks of endocrine cells within the islet. Most of the cells within these blocks are β-cells.

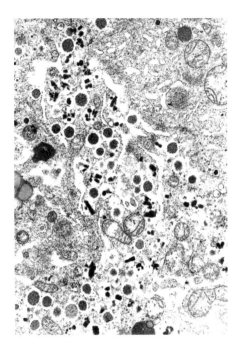

Figure 2.10 Electron micrograph of insulin storage granules (higher power view than in Figure 2.9) in a patient with an insulinoma.

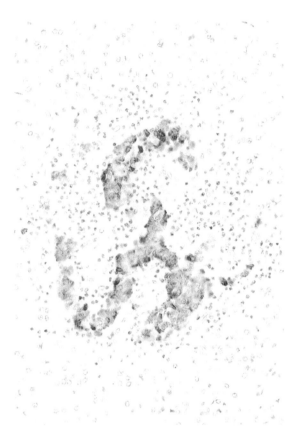

Figure 2.12 The same pancreas as in Figure 2.17 has been immunostained to show β-cells: note the destruction of the β-cells in this islet owing to inflammation; compare with Figure 2.6.

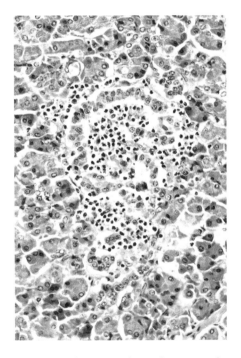

Figure 2.11 Insulitis. Histological section of a pancreas from a child who died at clinical presentation of type 1 diabetes mellitus. There is a heavy, chronic, inflammatory cell infiltrate affecting the islet. Haematoxylin and eosin stain.

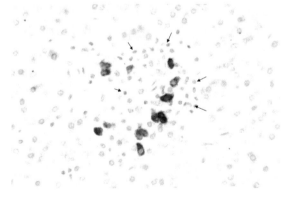

Figure 2.13 This histological section of pancreas was obtained at autopsy from a patient 5 years after the onset of type 1 diabetes mellitus (T1DM). It shows persistence of an infiltrate of lymphocytes (insulitis) some of which are indicated by arrows, affecting this islet, immunostained for insulin. This shows that β-cell destruction takes place over years in patients with T1DM.

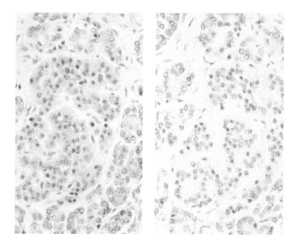

Figure 2.14 Autopsy section of an islet from a patient who had diabetes for 16 years. Although the islet looks fairly normal on haematoxylin and eosin stain (left), insulin staining (right) shows it is devoid of β-cells.

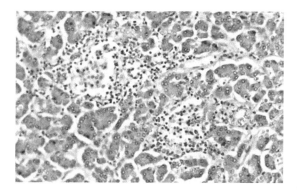

Figure 2.15 This is a section of pancreas from a 12-year-old boy who died of a cardiomyopathy. He had a family history of type 1 diabetes mellitus (T1DM) and was considered to be prediabetic because he had high titres of both insulin and islet cell autoantibodies in autopsy blood, but he did not have glycosuria in life. The photograph shows two islets affected by insulitis in his pancreas, confirming that immunologically mediated β-cell destruction takes place in the preclinical period of T1DM.

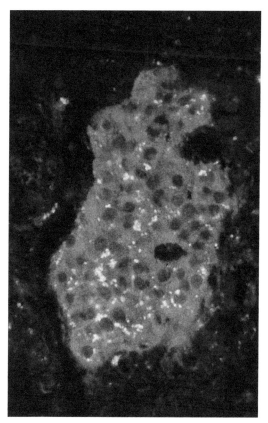

Figure 2.16 Circulating cytoplasmic islet-cell antibodies (ICA) can be found in most newly diagnosed type 1 diabetes mellitus (T1DM) patients, thereby providing evidence of an autoimmune pathogenesis of this disorder. ICA are also seen in the 'prediabetic' period and in siblings of T1DM patients, and are a marker of susceptibility to T1DM. This high-power view of a cryostat section of human pancreas was incubated with serum from a T1DM and stained by an indirect immunofluorescence technique using anti-human IgG fluorescinated antiserum. Although ICA are serological markers of β-cell destruction, the antibodies also stain the entire islet, including glucagon and somatostatin cells (which, unlike the β-cells, are not destroyed). The positive reaction is confined to cell cytoplasm and the nuclei are unstained (seen as black dots).

The rate of concordance is high in identical twins, but is much lower in non-identical dizygotic twins. Patients with T2DM show an increased frequency of diabetes in other family members compared with the non-diabetic population. Only a small proportion of patients (1–5%) with T2DM have a monogenic disorder (although this low percentage may reflect low diagnostic rates for monogenic diabetes). Obesity is the strongest risk factor for T2DM and there exists an inverse relationship between BMI and age of diagnosis of T2DM (although, of course, not all obese patients develop diabetes). It has been shown that a sedentary lifestyle is another risk factor for T2DM. Physical activity increases blood flow

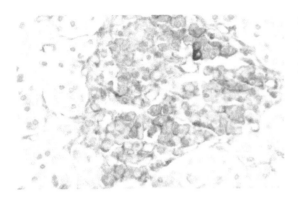

Figure 2.17 This section shows that all the endocrine cells (A, B, D, etc.) in this insulin-containing islet hyperexpress class 1 major histocompatibility complex (MHC). Note also that the islet is not inflamed (no lymphocytes). This suggests that hyperexpression of class 1 MHC precedes insulitis within any given islet and is not simply the result of secretion of cytokines by inflammatory cells in the insulitis infiltrate.

in skeletal muscles, thus increasing glucose uptake. It also reduces intra-abdominal fat, a key factor which promotes insulin resistance.

Pathogenesis of T2DM

Subjects with T2DM exhibit abnormalities in glucose homeostasis owing to impaired insulin secretion, insulin resistance in muscle, liver and adipocytes and abnormalities of splanchnic glucose uptake. The two cardinal features in terms of causation are defective insulin secretion by the pancreatic β-cells and an inability of normally insulin-sensitive tissues to respond to insulin.

Insulin secretion in T2DM

Impaired insulin secretion is a universal finding in patients with T2DM. In the early stages of T2DM, insulin resistance can be compensated for by an increase in insulin secretion, leading to normal glucose tolerance. With increasing insulin resistance, the fasting plasma glucose (FPG) will rise, accompanied by an increase in fasting plasma insulin levels, until an FPG level is reached when the β-cell is unable to maintain its elevated rate of insulin secretion, at which point the fasting plasma insulin declines sharply. When a state of excess nutrition exists, as in obesity, it will be accompanied by increased levels of free fatty acids (FFA) and hyperglycaemia. The resultant lipotoxicity and glucotoxicity induce metabolic and oxidative stress that leads to β-cell damage and signalling dysfunction. Sustained hyperglycaemia leads to the deposition of islet amyloid polypeptides (IAPP or amylin) which may further impair β-cell function. Hepatic glucose production will also begin to rise. When FPG reaches high levels, the plasma insulin response to a glucose challenge is markedly blunted. Although fasting insulin levels remain elevated, postprandial insulin and C-peptide secretory rates are decreased. This natural history of T2DM starting from normal glucose tolerance, followed by insulin resistance, compensatory hyperinsulinaemia and then by progression to impaired glucose tolerance (IGT) as a consequence of β-cell dysfunction and failure, as described previously, leading to overt diabetes, has been documented in a variety of populations (Figure 2.18).

T2DM is characterised by loss of the first-phase insulin response to an intravenous glucose load, although this abnormality may be acquired secondary to glucotoxicity. Loss of the first-phase insulin response is important as this early quick insulin secretion primes insulin target tissues, especially the liver.

There are multiple possible causes of the impaired insulin secretion in T2DM as alluded to previously, with several abnormalities having been shown to disturb the delicate balance between islet neogenesis and apoptosis. Studies in first-degree relatives of patients with T2DM and in twins have provided strong evidence for the genetic basis of abnormal β-cell function. Patients with T2DM also exhibit a reduced response of the incretin glucagon-like peptide-1 (GLP-1) in response to oral glucose, while GLP-1 administration enhances the postprandial insulin secretory response and may restore near-normal glycaemia. More recently, changes in the gut microbiota were implicated in the development of insulin resistance and T2DM but this area of research requires further exploration (Figure 2.19).

Insulin resistance in T2DM

Insulin resistance is a characteristic feature of both lean and obese individuals with T2DM and is described as a decrease in the metabolic response of insulin-sensitive cells to insulin.

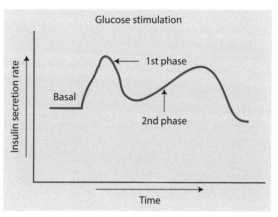

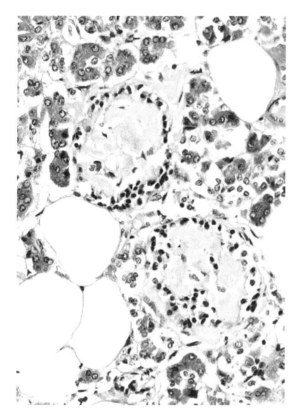

Figure 2.18 The characteristic histological abnormality in type 2 diabetes mellitus (T2DM) is amyloid deposition in the islets, which is significant in around two-thirds of cases. Increasing amounts of amyloid deposition are associated with progressive islet cell damage, which probably contributes to the insulin deficiency of T2DM. In this pancreas from a patient who had T2DM of long standing, two islets containing large deposits of amorphous pink-staining amyloid can be seen.

Skeletal muscle is the major site of insulin-stimulated glucose disposal in humans. Muscle represents the primary site of insulin resistance in T2DM subjects, leading to a marked blunting of glucose uptake into peripheral muscle. Mutations which reduce the expression of insulin receptor or the glucose transporter GLUT4 as well as any defects of the signalling pathway could reduce muscle glucose uptake leading to hyperglycaemia. Reduced physical activity decreases blood flow into muscle, thereby reducing muscle glucose uptake. Obesity has been associated with inflammatory changes in muscle impairing myocyte function, which could result in insulin resistance.

Figure 2.19 Biphasic insulin response to a constant glucose stimulus: when the β-cell is stimulated, there is a rapid first-phase insulin response 1–3 minutes after the glucose level is increased; this returns towards baseline 6–10 minutes later. Thereafter, there is a gradual second-phase insulin response that persists for the duration of the stimulus. Type 2 diabetes mellitus is characterized by loss of the first-phase insulin response and a diminished second-phase response.

In recent years adipose tissue has been recognised as an important metabolically dynamic tissue. An impaired response of adipose tissue to insulin constitutes adipose insulin resistance, whereby there is impaired suppression of lipolysis, impaired glucose uptake and enhanced FFA release into plasma. This results in hyperglycaemia and FFA accumulation in muscle, liver and the pancreas. Fat accumulation in the liver results in impaired insulin signalling that promotes increased hepatic glucose output via gluconeogenesis and impairs the glucose-stimulated insulin response. An increased adipose tissue mass leads to an increase in circulating proinflammatory molecules and the resultant chronic inflammatory state is considered to be a key element in the pathogenesis of insulin resistance. In summary, insulin resistance at hepatic level is associated with impaired glycogen synthesis, a failure to suppress glucose production, increased lipogenesis and a proinflammatory effect leading to glucotoxicity, lipotoxicity and a chronic inflammatory state. A high-calorie Western diet and reduced physical activity also contribute to chronic inflammation. There is increasing evidence that mitochondrial dysfunction may also be associated with insulin resistance and resultant T2DM. Splanchnic tissues, like the brain, are relatively insensitive to insulin with respect to stimulation of glucose uptake.

There is a dynamic relationship between insulin resistance and impaired insulin secretion. Insulin resistance is an early and characteristic feature of T2DM in high-risk populations. Overt diabetes develops only when the β-cells are unable to increase sufficiently their insulin output to compensate for the defect in insulin action (insulin resistance).

MONOGENIC AND OTHER TYPES OF DIABETES

The existence of a monogenic cause of diabetes in some cases was suspected by the observation of two main clinical phenotypes, namely, the onset of diabetes in neonates or infants (neonatal diabetes mellitus [NDM]) and families with several generations of diabetes occurring in adolescent or young adults suggesting an autosomal dominant mode of inheritance (maturity-onset diabetes of the young [MODY]). Other subtypes of monogenic diabetes exist and they include certain rare multisystem syndromes, cases of severe insulin resistance (in the absence of obesity) and patients with lipodystrophy (full or partial). The current approach is to define cases of monogenic diabetes based on molecular genetics. The current classification of monogenic diabetes combines the standard abbreviation of the gene involved followed by an accepted abbreviation of the clinical phenotype. An example of this would be GCK-MODY. The term MODY should not be confused with children or young adults presenting with true T2DM, a sadly increasing occurrence in Western and other societies. The most common causes of monogenic diabetes are listed in Figure 2.20.

Monogenic diabetes subtypes

GCK-MODY is characterised by a non-progressive hyperglycaemia and is the most common cause of monogenic diabetes with an estimated prevalence of 1 in 1000 individuals. GCK-MODY is caused by heterozygous inactivating mutations in the enzyme glucokinase, which acts as the β-cell glucose sensor. Impairment of GCK activity causes an increase in the threshold level of glucose required to initiate insulin secretion with the result being mild fasting hyperglycaemia of the order of

5.4–8.3 mmol/L (97–150 mg/dl) and a HbA_{1C} of 5.8–7.6% (40–60 mmol/mol). β-Cell function is otherwise normal. The abnormality is present from birth and remains stable. GCK-MODY is usually diagnosed incidentally and those affected are asymptomatic, require no treatment and exhibit no diabetic complications.

HNF1A-MODY and the less common HNF4A-MODY are caused by mutations in β-cell transcription factors with roles in the β-cell, liver and other organs. The importance of diagnosing these forms of monogenic diabetes is that the associated hyperglycaemia responds well to sulphonylurea treatment, thus obviating the need for other glucose-lowering drugs including insulin. HNFA4A MODY differs from HNF1A-MODY in that fetuses and newborn babies have excess insulin secretion leading to an excessive birth weight and possible macrosomia and neonatal hypoglycaemia. HNF1B-MODY is characterised by the presence of renal cysts with possible developmental abnormalities in multiple systems. Indeed, it is the commonest genetic causation of childhood kidney disease. HNF1B-MODY usually presents in adolescence or young adulthood and is frequently associated with reduced exocrine pancreatic function, which may require treatment.

KCNJ11-NDM and ABCC8-NDM are caused by activating heterozygous mutations in either gene encoding the subunits of the β-cell KATP channel and are the most common causes of permanent prenatal diabetes mellitus (PNDM) and NDM. Treatment with high doses of a sulphonylurea can reduce hyperglycaemia stably over many years. Neurodevelopmental abnormalities may coexist and be responsive to sulphonylurea treatment. Transient neonatal diabetes mellitus (TNDM) may be associated with overexpression of maternally methylated genes at chromosome 6q24 (imprinted locus at 6q24). Diabetes resolves spontaneously within the first year of life but usually recurs in adolescence or young adulthood, fortunately responding to oral agents.

Heterozygous mutations in the proinsulin gene (*INS*) produce *INS*-NDM and *INS*-MODY, the second most common cause of PNDM as a result of progressive loss of β-cell functional capacity due to accumulation of misfolded proinsulin protein. Affected individuals require insulin treatment. Multisystem syndromes caused by a single gene abnormality include mitochondrial diabetes and

Clinical implications of some common and important causes of monogenic diabetes

Gene	Inheritance/phenotypes	Disease mechanism/special features	Importance of genetic diagnosis
GCK	AD: GCK-MODY (common) AR: GCK-NDM (very rare)	Reduced function of glucokinase enzyme raises set point for insulin secretion that is otherwise normal; high population prevalence of causal variants (~1 in 1,000)	*No treatment needed* for most patients (except possibly during pregnancy)
HNF1A	AD: HNF1A-MODY (common)	LOF of β-cell transcription factor; glucosuria is common; risk for benign hepatic adenomas (rarely can become large and/or complicated)	Excellent glycemic control usually possible with low-dose oral sulfonylureas
HNF4A	AD: HNF4A-MODY (uncommon)	LOF of β-cell transcription factor; carriers may have history of large birth weights and/or hyperinsulinemic hypoglycemia	Often responsive to low-dose oral sulfonylureas
HNF1B	AD: HNF1B-MODY (uncommon)	LOF of pancreatic/renal transcription factor; renal cysts/genitourinary malformations (may be more penetrant than diabetes); hypomagnesemia; exocrine pancreatic insufficiency, altered liver function tests, hyperuricemia, developmental delay (as part of chromosome 17q deletion syndrome)	Optimal treatment for diabetes not well established; genetic diagnosis will inform monitoring and management of other features
ABCC8	AD/AR: ABCC8-NDM (common) ABCC8-MODY (rare)	Activating missense mutations in β-cell K_{ATP} channel SUR1 subunit impair glucose-stimulated insulin secretion; NDM may have a spectrum of neurodevelopmental dysfunction	Usually responds to high-dose oral sulfonylureas; genetic diagnosis facilitates monitoring/intervention for neurodevelopmental problems
KCNJ11	AD: KCNJ11-NDM (common) KCNJ11-MODY (rare)	Activating missense mutations in β-cell K_{ATP} channel Kir6.2 subunit impair glucose-stimulated insulin secretion; NDM often have a spectrum of neurodevelopmental dysfunction	Usually responds to high-dose oral sulfonylureas; genetic diagnosis facilitates monitoring/intervention for neurodevelopmental problems
6q24 (imprinted locus)	Most common cause of transient NDM	Overexpression of maternally imprinted 6q24 genes causes impairment of β-cell development and function; after remission of NDM within first year of life, diabetes will often recur in adolescence or adulthood	Diabetes recurring later in life is often responsive to noninsulin therapies
INS	AD/AR: INS-NDM (common) AD: INS-MODY (rare)	Missense mutations cause insulin protein misfolding and progressive β-cell death (other mechanisms occur more rarely)	Early intensive insulin treatment; future treatments may feasibly target molecular mechanism(s)

AD, autosomal dominant; AR, autosomal recessive; Kir6.2, inward rectifier potassium channel 6.2; SUR, sulfonylurea receptor.

Figure 2.20 Clinical implications of some common and important causes of monogenic diabetes.

Wolfram syndrome. Mitochondrial diabetes is associated with sensorineural deafness and other possible renal, cardiac and neurological features while Wolfram syndrome features sensorineural deafness, optic atrophy and diabetes insipidus and is usually caused by recessive mutations in *WFS1*.

As previously described, diabetes may result from overt diseases of the exocrine pancreas, secondary to specific endocrinopathies and due to drugs or chemicals. Certain viruses have been associated with β-cell destruction (coxsackievirus B, cytomegalovirus, adenovirus, mumps, congenital rubella), although, in most cases, the precise nature of the association remains unclear. Many other genetic syndromes are accompanied by an increased incidence of diabetes (Down's syndrome, Klinefelter's syndrome, Turner's syndrome, Prader-Willi syndrome) (Figures 2.21–2.37).

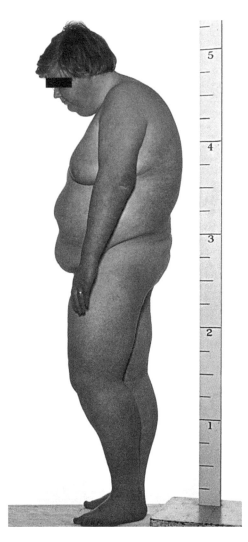

Figure 2.21 Prader-Willi syndrome is a syndrome of obesity, muscular hypotonia, hypogonadotropic hypogonadism and mental retardation associated, in about 50% of cases, with a deletion or translocation of chromosome 15. A small percentage of patients have type 2 diabetes mellitus.

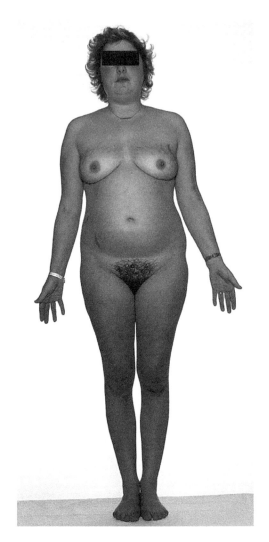

Figure 2.22 The centripetal obesity and prominent lipid striae suggest that this is Cushing's syndrome and not simple obesity.

THE OBESITY EPIDEMIC

A dramatic increase in the prevalence of obesity has been witnessed in many countries in the past quarter of a century. Obesity, at least in Caucasian populations, is defined as a body mass index (BMI; weight [kg]/height [m]^2) >30. In South Asian populations, a BMI >23 is associated with an increased health risk while a BMI >25 is defined as obesity. This is because these populations have an increased body fat content at a given BMI compared to Caucasian populations. BMI is not a direct measurement of body fat but is moderately correlated with body fat measured directly. BMI may not accurately reflect fat mass nor its distribution in some individuals, particularly high-level athletes. Fairly accurate estimations of fat distribution may be gained by measuring the waist–hip ratio or more simply waist circumference, both of which correlate well with more sophisticated techniques, such as computed tomography or magnetic resonance imaging. Weight-related health problems are more common in males with a waist circumference greater than 102 cm (40 inches) and in females with a waist circumference greater than

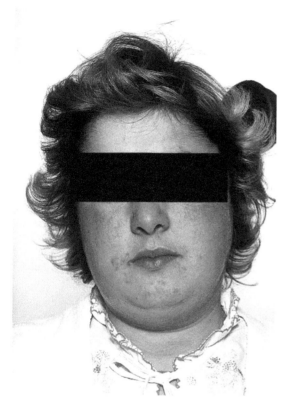

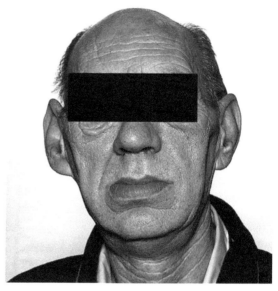

Figure 2.24 Diabetes occurs in 15–30% of patients with acromegaly and similarly with impaired glucose tolerance. The excess growth hormone secretion, usually from a pituitary adenoma, is associated with insulin resistance which, after several years, may result in the diabetic state. The diabetes is usually type 2, and is associated with the usual microvascular and other complications. Glucose tolerance improves after successful treatment of the acromegaly.

Figure 2.23 This young woman (same patient as in Figure 2.22) has the typical facies of Cushing's syndrome—a rounded plethoric face and mild hirsutism. Glucose tolerance is impaired in most patients with Cushing's syndrome and about 25% of patients are diabetic. However, many older patients with type 2 diabetes mellitus have features of Cushing's syndrome, specifically, obesity, hirsutism, hypertension, striae and diabetes, but do not have the condition.

89 cm (35 inches). The measurement of waist circumference has become part of the definition of the metabolic syndrome, a condition associated with vascular risk factors and which predisposes to the development of T2DM. The overall prevalence of obesity in the UK was 28% in 2022, while as of 2020 it was 42% in the US (even higher in the Non-Hispanic Black population). One in seven children in the UK are obese by the age of 5 years and one in four by the age of 11 years. Childhood obesity is particularly present in deprived areas. At 2018 in the US, one in five children and adolescents between 2 and 19 years of age were obese. In England, the adult prevalence of obesity increased by 15% between 1993 and 2019, with similar or

greater trends elsewhere. It is estimated that 12% of the world population is obese, a tripling in prevalence since 1975. Although there is a suggestion that the rate of increase in obesity is declining in high-income countries, it continues to increase in low-income and middle-income countries. People of all ages, races, ethnicities, socioeconomic levels and geographical areas are experiencing a substantial increase in weight. Such data have led to the coining of the term 'the obesity epidemic', sometimes stated as 'the obesity pandemic', as this problem is not confined to the developed nations of the world but is also happening in developing nations, particularly in affluent strata of society.

Food intake

It is clear that obesity results from the interaction of many factors including genetic, metabolic, behavioural and environmental influences, but the

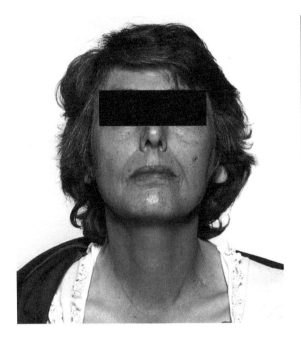

Figure 2.25 About 10% of patients with Addison's disease have diabetes, usually type 1. Diabetic patients who develop Addison's disease exhibit an increased sensitivity to insulin which is reversed by glucocorticoid replacement therapy. Addison's disease and associated type 1 diabetes mellitus or other autoimmune endocrinopathy (such as hypothyroidism, Graves' disease and hypoparathyroidism) is referred to as Schmidt's syndrome.

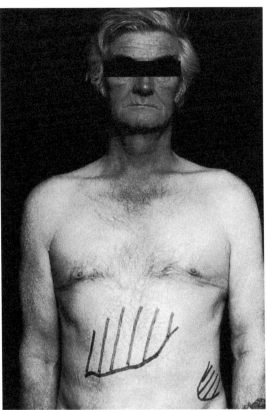

Figure 2.26 This patient has hereditary haemochromatosis transmitted by an autosomal recessive gene. It occurs most commonly as a result of a mutation in the gene *HFE*—on the short arm of chromosome 6. Patients present with the classic triad of bronze skin pigmentation, hepatomegaly and diabetes mellitus (hence the term 'bronze diabetes'). Cardiac manifestations and pituitary dysfunction also occur.

rapidity with which obesity is increasing, in the context of a relatively stable gene pool, suggests that environmental and behavioural factors largely explain the epidemic. National trends in food consumption have revealed conflicting data; however, ecological data seem to support the notion that energy intake has increased perhaps related to an increased percentage of food consumed outside the home including fast foods, greater consumption of soft drinks and larger portion sizes.

Energy expenditure

Although it is difficult to quantify, it seems likely that a major downward change in physical activity and, thus, energy expenditure, plays a significant role in the development of obesity in modern society whether or not energy intake has increased. This includes the level of activity required at work and in the home, reduced dependence on walking and cycling for transportation, reduced physical

activity in schools and more jobs being of a sedentary nature. In the US, 15% (range 17.3–47.7) of the population was described as physically inactive, defined as not participating in any leisure-time physical activities in the last month, while in the UK, 25% of people over the age of 16 years were physically inactive, defined as taking less than 30 minutes of moderate-intensity physical activities per week. A cross-sectional study in South Carolina, US, suggested that obese children spent less time in moderate and vigorous physical activity than their non-obese counterparts, and in a national US study, children who engaged in the least vigorous physical activity or the most television viewing tended to be the most overweight.

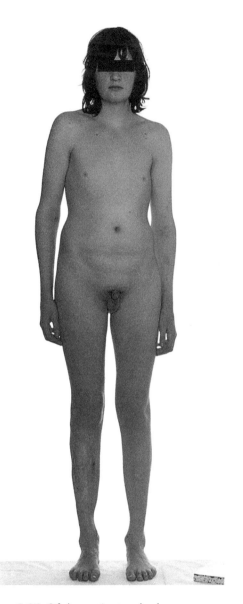

Figure 2.27 Of the patients who have Klinefelter's syndrome (47,XXY karyotype), 26% show diabetes on the oral glucose tolerance test, but overt symptomatic diabetes is unusual. The cause of the diabetes is not known, but may be related to insulin resistance.

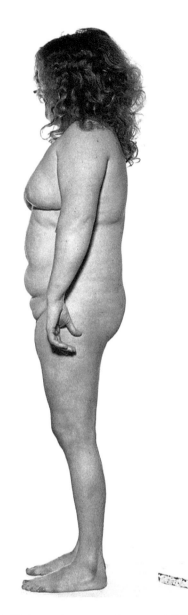

Figure 2.28 Diabetes is present in around 60% of young adults with Turner's syndrome (45,XO karyotype) and is usually type 2. A paradoxical rise in growth hormone to oral glucose may be the cause of the glucose intolerance.

Genetics and obesity

From a genetic viewpoint, obesity may be considered either rare, early-onset and severe monogenic obesity or polygenic (common obesity), although it is likely that there is overlap between the two phenotypes. Gene discoveries suggest that the central nervous system and neuronal pathways controlling the hedonistic aspects of food intake are the main drivers of obesity in both monogenic and polygenic obesity. The genes for leptin, a hormone produced by fat which reduces energy intake, and its receptor became candidates for obesity. In 1997, congenital leptin deficiency was identified leading to obesity and this discovery was followed by identification of genes encoding the leptin receptor

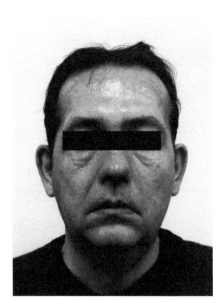

Figure 2.29 The typical facies of myotonic dystrophy, with frontal balding and a smooth forehead, is associated, albeit rarely, with diabetes mellitus. Impaired glucose tolerance with insulin resistance is more commonly found.

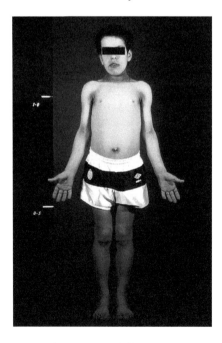

Figure 2.30 This 13-year-old boy with Rabson–Mendenhall syndrome exhibits severe insulin resistance (moderate hyperglycaemia associated with gross elevation of plasma insulin levels). Typically associated features include stunted growth and acanthosis nigricans, affecting the neck, axillae and antecubital fossae, and a characteristic facies.

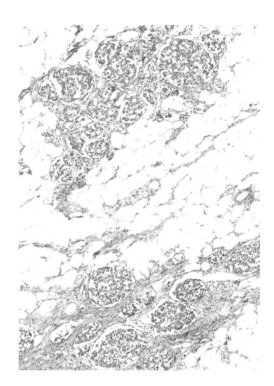

Figure 2.31 Glucose intolerance occurs in about 30% of cases of cystic fibrosis, although only 1–2% of patients have frank diabetes. This low-power view of the pancreas of a 14-year-old child with cystic fibrosis complicated by diabetes shows complete atrophy of the exocrine pancreas, but with survival of the islets. Some of the islets (lower part of field) are embedded in fibrous tissue. Haematoxylin and eosin stain.

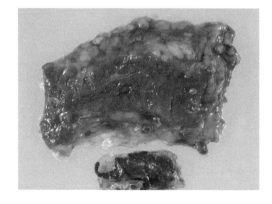

Figure 2.32 This is a coronal section of the tail of the pancreas from a patient with haemochromatosis. Note the brown colour of the pancreas compared with the surrounding fat. Normal pancreas tissue appears pale. The smaller piece of pancreas has been stained with Prussian blue to show the presence of iron deposits.

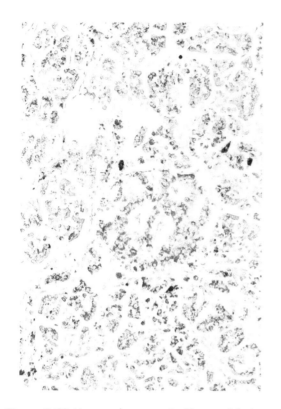

Figure 2.33 Haemochromatosis. Haemosiderin deposits in this low-power view of pancreas are stained blue. Note the accumulation of iron in the endocrine cells of the islet (centre) as well as in the acinar cells of the exocrine pancreas. Prussian blue staining was used.

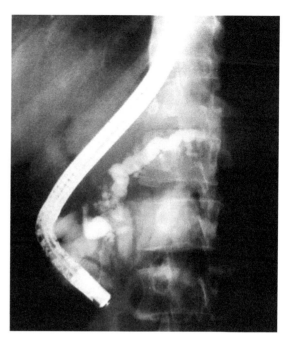

Figure 2.35 This endoscopic retrograde cholan-giopancreato-gram shows the typical appear-ances of chronic pancreatitis. There is a dilated pancreatic duct with amputation and beading of the side branches.

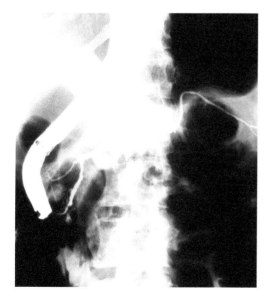

Figure 2.34 This endoscopic retrograde cholangi-opancreato-gram shows a normal pancreatic duct.

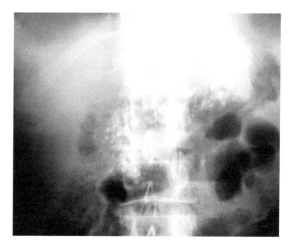

Figure 2.36 Plain abdominal radiograph show-ing pancreatic calcification due to chronic pancreatitis. Diabetes occurs in around 45% of cases of chronic pancreatitis and is usually mild. Approximately one-third of patients will ultimately require insulin treatment to maintain adequate glycaemic control.

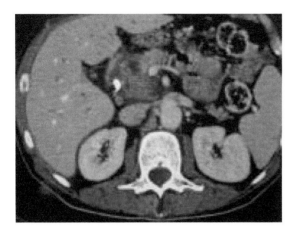

Figure 2.37 This computed tomography scan shows cancer of the pancreas. An association between adenocarcinoma of the pancreas and diabetes has long been recognized. Pancreatic cancer may precede the diagnosis of diabetes, but some epidemiological studies suggest that there is an increased risk of pancreatic cancer in diabetic patients. Unexplained weight loss or back pain in a patient with type 2 diabetes mellitus must always raise the suspicion of underlying pancreatic cancer.

as well as genes encoding multiple components of the melanocortin pathway, all of which were found to result in severe early-onset obesity. Other monogenic obesity mutations have been identified. GWAS are ongoing, but variants in only six genes show reproducible association with obesity outcomes. Nevertheless, such studies are likely to deliver knowledge about the relationship between gene defects and the 'obesogenic' environment.

Sequelae of obesity

Obesity is associated with an increased risk of heart disease, hypertension, a variety of cancers, cerebrovascular disease, gallstones and osteoarthritis; furthermore, it has also been associated with an alarming increase in the prevalence of T2DM with adults presenting at an ever-earlier age and the disturbing appearance of T2DM in adolescents and children. The health and economic consequences of this are likely to be devastating, thus, the obesity epidemic has to be considered a global issue of major importance. Governments and their politicians must address this issue and develop workable public health policies and legislation to reverse the obesity trend (Figures 2.38 and 2.39).

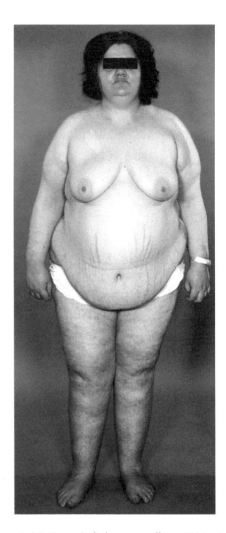

Figure 2.38 Type 2 diabetes mellitus (T2DM) is strongly associated with obesity and this link has been recognized for centuries. The risk of developing T2DM increases progressively with rising body mass index. T2DM is the result of increased insulin resistance and insulin deficiency. Obesity is strongly associated with insulin resistance and high fasting insulin levels. It has been proposed that this may ultimately result in β-cell failure and the emergence of T2DM; however, this theory is oversimplistic and the precise cause of T2DM remains unknown except in a few cases of identified genetic abnormalities.

PREVENTION OF DIABETES

T1DM

Prevention of the loss of β-cell mass is a major challenge in T1DM research. On the basis of the theory that immune-mediated T1DM is believed to result

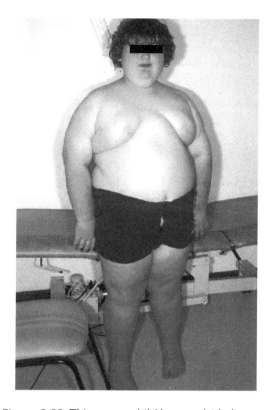

Figure 2.39 This young child has morbid obesity. As the age of peak incidence of diabetes declines, cases of type 2 diabetes mellitus are now being identified in such children and in young adolescents, especially in highly susceptible ethnic groups. The health consequences of this phenomenon are likely to be immense.

from immunological destruction of islet β-cells as a consequence of an interplay between genetic susceptibility and a triggering environmental agent or agents, it would seem possible to identify potential targets for prevention of the disease, although we know that the previously discussed theory is very much an oversimplification of the true pathological mechanism. The development of T1DM is a slow process with the best prospect of preventive strategies occurring early in the disease process. At that stage, disease prediction is less accurate and any treatment would need to be safe, otherwise, individuals may be harmed by a treatment who were never going to develop the disease. Strategies to prevent T1DM would include (a) identification and elimination of environmental triggers, (b) identification and promotion of environmental protective factors and (c) interruption of the immunological process leading to β-cell destruction. A target population for preventative trials would be those

who have a high-risk genotype plus or minus the presence of islet autoantibodies. Low-risk dietary intervention trials in genetically susceptible individuals without autoantibodies have been largely unsuccessful (NIP, DAISY, TRIGR, FINDIA, BABYDIET, Diabetes TrialNet).

Trials using the administration of nicotinamide, which can prevent T1DM in animal models, have failed to prevent diabetes as have trials of insulin administration using the oral, nasal or subcutaneous route. Immunotherapy with monoclonal antibodies (for example, teplizumab which targets CD8 lymphocytes) holds the greatest promise in T1DM prevention. The T1DM TrialNet Study Group trial demonstrated for the first time that treatment with teplizumab delayed the onset of T1DM in a high-risk group by a median of 2 years. Teplizumab has also been trialled in patients with established T1DM where is has been shown to be effective in preserving C-peptide secretion when administered early in the course of the disease. Other agents that have been used in tertiary prevention are cyclosporine A and azathioprine with glucocorticoids. These have shown an effect on preservation of insulin secretion in some individuals but, unfortunately, the effect was not prolonged. Treatment of new-onset T1DM patients with a class of immunosuppressive lymphocytes known as regulatory T cells (Tregs) can delay β-cell destruction. Monoclonal antibodies and other immune-modifying agents would seem to hold out the best promise as preventative agents in T1DM. There may be a role for vaccines but such research is at an early stage.

T2DM

Expanding prevalence rates of T2DM diabetes both in developed and developing nations dictate that the prevention of T2DM is an issue of global importance. Clearly the prevention of T2DM is closely related to the prevention of obesity. T2DM lends itself to potential preventative action because of the long delay between development of the earliest metabolic defects and full expression of the disease. Lifestyle modification (weight loss and increased physical activity) is without doubt the most effective way to prevent progression to frank diabetes. Lifestyle modification or pharmacological intervention that can improve insulin sensitivity (reduce insulin resistance) or improve or preserve β-cell function would be expected to have an impact on the future development of T2DM.

The first major trial to show the effect of lifestyle change on the development of diabetes was the Da Qing Study in China where patients with IGT were randomised to a control group and one of three active treatment groups (change in diet, exercise or change in diet plus exercise). The diet group experienced a relative risk reduction of progression to frank diabetes of 31%, the exercise group of 46% and the combined group of 42%. Follow-up data revealed a 39% reduction in diabetes at 30 years.

This study was followed by the Finnish Diabetes Prevention Study, which compared lifestyle intervention to a control group in overweight patients with IGT. The lifestyle intervention group received detailed dietary advice and individualised advice on physical activity with supervised training sessions. During the first year of the study, the intervention group achieved a significant loss of 4.2 kg with minimal change in the control group and after 2 years, the cumulative incidence of progression to diabetes was reduced by 58%. Whether such an intensity of lifestyle intervention could be provided, funded and adhered to outside the context of a clinical trial remains open to debate. However, the investigators reported a 43% reduction in new diabetes cases after 7 years of follow-up.

In the US, the investigators in the Diabetes Prevention Program randomly assigned patients with IGT to one of three arms: placebo, lifestyle modification or metformin (850 mg twice daily). Patients in the lifestyle intervention group were asked to achieve and maintain a reduction of at least 7% in body weight through a healthy diet and to engage in moderate physical activity for at least 150 minutes per week. Patients received intensive support and, as for the Finnish study, such a level of support is unlikely to be available in routine clinical practice. The lifestyle group achieved a greater weight loss (5.6 kg) and a greater increase in physical activity than the other groups. At 3 years, the prevalence of T2DM was reduced by 58% with lifestyle change and by 31% in the metformin group. After 15 years of follow-up, diabetes incidence was reduced by 27% by lifestyle intervention. Accordingly, The American Diabetes Association (ADA) recommends intensive lifestyle modification for the prevention of diabetes in patients with 'prediabetes' and states that metformin therapy should be recommended for those at high risk of developing T2DM (previous history of gestational diabetes mellitus or BMI greater than or equal to 35).

The multinational Study to Prevent Non-Insulin Dependent Diabetes Mellitus (STOP-NIDDM Trial) used acarbose to prevent progression to diabetes in IGT subjects. Patients who were randomised to acarbose were 25% less likely to develop diabetes, and when the data were corrected to the current ADA criteria for the diagnosis of diabetes, there was an even greater relative risk reduction of 32%. Treatment with a glitazone has also been shown to reduce the number of patients who develop diabetes 30 months after gestational diabetes with a 55% relative risk reduction in the Troglitazone in Prevention of Diabetes (TRIPOD) study, although troglitazone is no longer available, and the use of pioglitazone in subjects with IGT in the Assessing the Effectiveness of Communication Therapy in the North West (ACTNOW) study reduced the conversion to T2DM by 72%, while 42% of the pioglitazone subjects reverted to normal glucose tolerance.

Several other T2DM pharmacological prevention trials have been conducted. In the Trial of Prevention of Cardiovascular Complications and Type 2 Diabetes with Valsartan and/or Nateglinide (NAVIGATOR) study, the use of nateglinide was not associated with any reduction in diabetes incidence or cardiovascular outcomes. Subjects in the DREAM (Diabetes Reduction Assessment with Ramipril and Rosiglitazone Medication) study with IFG or IGT were treated with ramipril for 3 years with no significant decrease in diabetes incidence or death (although there was a significant increase in the number of individuals regressing to normoglycaemia). In the Outcome Reduction with Initial Glargine (ORIGIN) study, people with cardiovascular risk factors and IFG, IGT or T2DM were treated with an injection of basal insulin glargine. This had a neutral effect on cardiovascular outcomes and cancer cases but reduced new onset diabetes (30% vs. 35% 3 months after glargine stopped) but with an increase in hypoglycaemia and an increase in weight.

Thus, it has been conclusively shown that lifestyle modification and drug therapy can delay the onset of T2DM. Whether there has been true 'prevention' in those subjects who did not develop diabetes is a different matter, and it may seem counterintuitive to prevent diabetes by the use of agents to treat diabetes. Cost-effective analyses would also have to be taken into consideration, although individual health benefit is likely to ensue.

Reversal of T2DM

Prolonged excess calorie intake leads to fat accumulation in the liver. Increased liver fat causes relative resistance to hepatic glucose production by insulin. The resultant increase in FPG leads to hyperinsulinaemia, which further increases the conversion of excess calories into liver fat. A fatty liver results in excess export of very low-density-lipoprotein (VLDL) triacylglycerol increasing fat delivery to the pancreatic islets, which impairs the acute insulin secretion to ingested food resulting in postprandial hyperglycaemia. This results in a further increase in insulin secretion and further augmentation of liver and pancreatic islet fat deposition in a vicious cycle, the end result being the emergence of diabetes. This is known as the twin cycle hypothesis. The Counterpoint study showed that patients diagnosed with T2DM within 4 years who adhered to a very low-calorie liquid diet (600 kcal) for 8 weeks while carrying on a normal life and who lost on average 15 kg in weight, exhibited a fall to normal levels of previously high levels of liver and pancreatic fat and decreased their hepatic glucose output and improved their β-cell function. Seventy-three percent achieved remission of T2DM. Subsequent studies (Counterbalance, Diabetes Remission Clinical Trial [DiRECT]) confirmed these findings, although remission rates are lower for patients with longer duration of diabetes. The importance of these studies is the knowledge that, for some people, T2DM may be reversible even when severe calorie restriction is relaxed.

BIBLIOGRAPHY

Andersen RE, Crespo CJ, Bartlett SJ, et al. Relationship of physical activity and television watching with body weight and level of fatness among children: results from the third national health and nutrition examination survey. JAMA. 1998; 279: 938–42

Atkinson MA, Eisenbarth GS. Type I diabetes: new perspectives on disease pathogenesis and treatment. Lancet. 2001; 358: 221–9

Beik P, Ciesielska M, et al. Prevention of type 1 diabetes: past experience and future opportunities. J Clin Med. 2020 Sep; 9(9): 2805. Doi: 10.3390/jcm9092805

Besser R, Ng SM, Robertson EJ. Screening children for type 1 diabetes. BMJ 2021; 375: e067937. Doi: 10.1136/bmj-2021-067937

Bottazzo GF. Death of a beta cell: homicide or suicide? Diabetic Med. 1986; 3: 119–30

Chiasson JL, Gomis R, Hanefeld M, et al. The STOP-NIDDM trial: an international study on the efficacy of an alpha-glucosidase inhibitor to prevent type 2 diabetes in a population with impaired glucose tolerance: rationale, design, and preliminary screening data. Study to prevent non-insulin-dependent Diabetes Mellitus. Diabetes Care. 1998; 21: 1720–5

DeFronzo R. The triumvirate: β-cell, muscle, liver. a collusion responsible for NIDDM. Diabetes. 1988; 37: 667–75

DeFronzo RA. Pathogenesis of type 2 diabetes mellitus. Med Clin North Am. 2004; 88: 787–835

Ebbeling CB, Pawiak DB, Ludwig DS. Childhood obesity: public-health crisis, common sense cure. Lancet. 2002; 360: 473–82

Froguel P, Velho G. Genetic determinants of type 2 diabetes. Recent Prog Horm Res. 2001; 56: 91–105

Fujimoto WY. The importance of insulin resistance in the pathogenesis of type 2 diabetes mellitus. Am J Med. 2000; 108(Suppl 6a): 9s–14s

Giwa AM, Ahmed R, Omidian Z, et al. Current understandings of the pathogenesis of type 1 diabetes: genetics to environment. World J Diabetes. 2020 Jan 15; 11(1): 13–25. Doi: 10.4239/wjd.v11.i1.13

Hitman GA. The major histocompatibility complex and insulin dependent (type I) diabetes. Autoimmunity. 1989; 4: 119–30

Inzucchi SE, Sherwin RS. The prevention of type 2 diabetes mellitus. Endocrinol Metab Clin North Am. 2005; 34: 199–219

Kahn SE. The importance of the beta-cell in the pathogenesis of type 2 diabetes mellitus. Am J Med. 2000; 108(Suppl 6a): 2s–8s

Krischer JP, Liu X, Lernmark A, et al. The influence of type 1 diabetes genetic susceptibility regions, age, sex and family history to the progression from multiple autoantibodies to type 1 diabetes: a TEDDY study report. Diabetes. 2017.66 3122–29. Doi: 10.2337/db17-0261

Paschou SA, Papadopoulou-Marketou N, Chrousos GP, et al. On type 1 diabetes mellitus pathogenesis. Endocr Connect. 2018 Jan; 7(1): R38–R46. Doi: 10.1530/EC-17-0347

Redondo MJ, Fain PR, Eisenbarth GS. Genetics of type IA diabetes. Recent Prog Horm Res. 2001; 56: 69–89

Riddle MC, Philipson LH, Rich SS, et al. Monogenic diabetes: from genetic insights to population-based precision in care. Reflections from a diabetes care Editors' expert forum. Diabetes Care. 2020; 43(12): 3117–28. Doi.org/10.2337/dci20-0065

Skyler JS. Immunotherapy for interdicting the type 1 diabetes disease process. In Pickup J, Williams G, eds. Textbook of Diabetes, 3rd edn. Oxford: Blackwell Scientific Publications, 2003: 74.1–74.12

Trost SG, Kerr LM, Ward DS, Pate RR. Physical activity and determinates of physical activity in obese and non-obese children. Int J Obes Relat Metab Disord. 2001; 25: 822–9

Taylor R. Calorie restriction for long-term remission of type 2 diabetes. Clin Med (Lond). 2019 Jan; 19(1): 37–42. Doi: 10.7861/clinmedicine.19-1-37

Undlien DE, Lie BA, Thorsby E. HLA complex genes in type I diabetes and other autoimmune diseases. Which genes are involved? Trends Genet. 2001; 17: 93–100

Zimmet PZ. The pathogenesis and prevention of diabetes in adults. Genes, autoimmunity, and demography. Diabetes Care. 1995; 18: 1050–64

3

Treatment of type 1 diabetes mellitus

INTRODUCTION

Effective treatment of type 1 diabetes mellitus (T1DM) first became possible with the introduction of insulin to clinical practice in 1922. Initial insulin preparations were variable in strength and were short acting, requiring repeated dosing with meals. In 1936, the first long-acting insulin was produced combining insulin with protamine and zinc to create a product that was absorbed slowly after subcutaneous injection to enable maintenance of blood insulin levels over the course of the day. As a result, it became possible to offer more physiological insulin replacement combining a long-acting 'basal' insulin to replace basal insulin secretion with a mealtime 'bolus' to mimic the rise in insulin occurring in the postprandial state. Various pre-mixed insulins were produced, combining variable proportions of short- and long-acting insulins, and the majority of people with T1DM were managed on two injections a day with occasional urine or blood glucose testing, with the aim of maintaining moderate control of glucose and avoiding acute metabolic decompensation. Challenges with early insulin treatment included local issues at injection sites including lipoatrophy, which was more commonly observed with animal sequence insulin than with modern insulins.

The need for a more intensive approach and the importance of maintaining tight blood glucose control in T1DM was established beyond doubt following the publication of the Diabetes Control and Complications Trial (DCCT) in 1993. This study enrolled more than 1400 patients with T1DM aged between 13 and 39 years of which half had no diabetes complications and half had evidence of retinopathy or microalbuminuria. Patients were randomised to a 'conventional' regime based on standard practice at the time (typically one or two daily injections) or an 'intensive' treatment regime comprising three or more insulin injections a day and four times daily blood glucose testing. A subgroup of the 'intensive' treatment arm used the then-new technology of continuous subcutaneous insulin delivery by insulin pump.

The difference in outcomes were striking. After 6.4 years of follow-up, the intensive group achieved a mean HbA_{1C} of 7% (53 mmol/mol) compared to 9% (76 mmol/mol) in the conventional group. This difference was associated with a 76% reduction in new retinopathy and a 50–60% reduction in onset or progression of diabetic nephropathy and neuropathy. Long-term follow-up of the cohort of patients who participated in the DCCT has shown that the benefits observed were sustained for more than 20 years with substantially lower rates of nephropathy and retinopathy in the intensively managed group and with one-third lower mortality in these patients when compared to those who received conventional treatment.

On the basis of these results, subsequent T1DM guidelines have evolved to recommend very tight blood glucose control and to aim for near normoglycaemia with recommended targets for HbA_{1C} ranging from 48 to 53 mmol/mol (6.5% to 7.0%). Despite such guidance and advancements in the management of diabetes, the majority of patients continue to have suboptimal control. In the UK, only 9.8% of adults with T1DM achieved a HbA_{1C} under 48 mmol/mol and only 19.5% achieved a value under 53 mmol/l, with some 14.4% having values above 86 mmol/mol, a cut-off selected to identify a very high-risk population.

These data reflect the challenges of managing diabetes in adults with T1DM. Significant barriers remain to optimising control, particularly

DOI: 10.1201/9781003342700-3

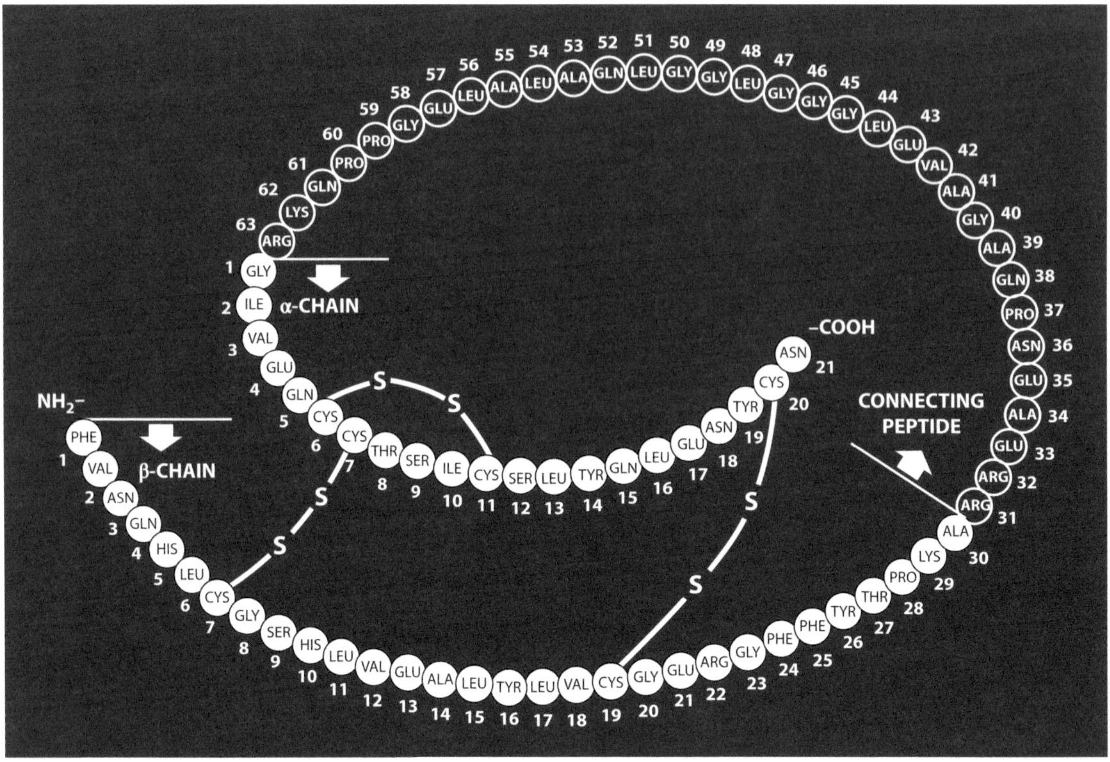

Figure 3.1 The structure of human proinsulin. Insulin is produced in the β-cells of the islets of Langerhans by cleavage of the precursor proinsulin into insulin and C-peptide. Measurement of C-peptide, especially following intravenous injection of 1 mg of glucagon, is a useful indicator of β-cell function, as C-peptide and insulin are secreted in equimolar amounts and the former is minimally extracted by the liver. This test can be used to differentiate between types 1 and 2 diabetes mellitus in cases of diagnostic confusion.

in relation to avoidance of hypoglycaemia and to managing the burden of living with T1DM on a continuing basis. However, there are ongoing developments that continue to improve the management of T1DM (Figures 3.1–3.7).

DEVELOPMENT OF INSULIN PREPARATIONS

At the time of the DCCT, the range of available insulins was limited and there have been significant advances in insulin biochemistry since then with the development of insulin analogues with different rates of absorption from subcutaneous tissue which can allow for differing durations of actions and properties.

For mealtime bolus delivery, the only available insulins then were soluble human or porcine

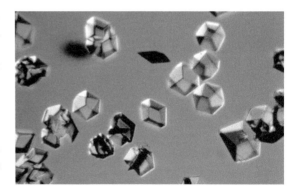

Figure 3.2 Insulin crystals. Insulin is stored in β-cells as hexamers complexed with zinc. Insulin–zinc hexamers readily form crystals, which are stored in the pancreatic granules. Following subcutaneous injection, insulin similarly tends to self-aggregate into hexamers but needs to dissociate into its monomeric form to enter the blood.

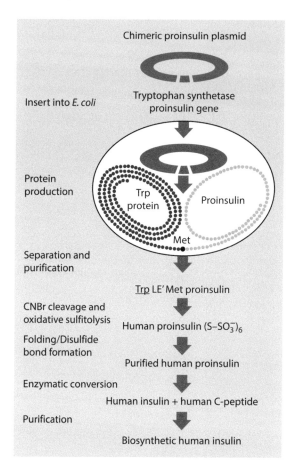

Figure 3.3 Insulin for therapeutic use was previously produced solely from porcine or bovine sources. Nearly all insulin now used is produced by biosynthesis of human sequence insulin and analogues created by further amino acid substitution and in some cases, addition of fatty acid chains to prolong action. Porcine and human insulin differ only in a single residue at the C terminus of the β chain. Enzymatic conversion involves substitution of the porcine B30 alanine residue by threonine to produce the semisynthetic human insulin enzymatically modified porcine ('emp'). The biosynthesis of human insulin using recombinant-DNA technology involves insertion of a synthetic gene coding for human proinsulin into a bacterial plasmid, which is then introduced into a bacterium such as *Escherichia coli*. Ultimately, the synthetic gene is transcribed in quantity and its messenger RNA translated into proinsulin.

sequence insulin, which, while similar to native insulin in amino acid structure, did have significant variability in absorption after subcutaneous injection. This is due to the natural properties of

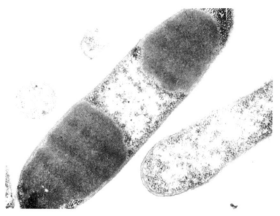

Figure 3.4 *Escherichia coli* distended by biosynthetic human proinsulin before lysis.

insulin molecules to combine to form hexamers; following subcutaneous injection, these hexamers need to dissociate into monomers to enable absorption into the circulation and this occurs at a variable rate. Since then, two new insulin analogues insulin aspart and insulin lispro have been developed with amino acid substitutions that result in the insulin mainly existing as dimers rather than hexamers, resulting in more rapid insulin absorption into the circulation and a more predictable postprandial glucose response.

For basal insulin replacement, the DCCT patients predominantly used isophane insulins. These have an effective duration of action of 12–16 hours, but a pronounced peak in insulin levels occurring at around 6–8 hours, which, for some patients, could lead to hypoglycaemia between meals or overnight. In T1DM treatment, these have now largely been replaced by long-acting insulin analogues with more predictable absorption and absence of peaks. The first-generation basal analogues insulin glargine (marketed as Lantus and its biosimilar Abasaglar) and insulin detemir (Levemir) were introduced shortly after the millennium and were associated with less hypoglycaemia (particularly nocturnal hypoglycaemia) compared to isophane insulin preparations. However, they still required twice-daily dosing for optimal basal insulin replacement. A second generation of basal insulin analogues has since appeared, comprising insulin degludec (Tresiba) and Toujeo, a concentrated preparation of insulin glargine. Both of these insulins have effective actions greater than 24 hours and, as a result,

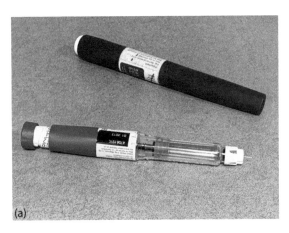 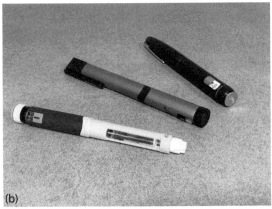

Figure 3.5 Almost all conventional insulin treatment is provided by the use of insulin 'pens'. These were first introduced in the mid-1980s and include fully disposable devices such as the Lilly Kwikpen® and Novo Nordisk 'Flexpen®' (a) and reusable robust devices that take 3 ml pre-filled insulin cartridges such as the Lilly Humapen® and Novo Nordisk Novopen® (b). Recently, new 'smart' insulin pens have been introduced that record data on insulin dose administration with the potential to link via Bluetooth technology to diabetes management apps.

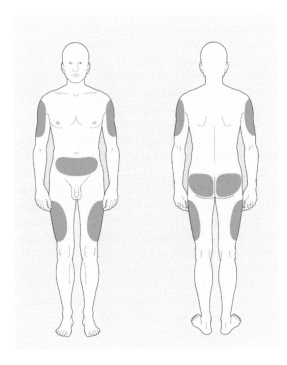

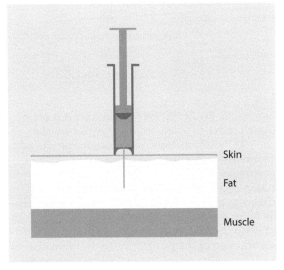

Figure 3.7 Insulin injection technique: The modern practice is to insert the needle vertically into the subcutaneous tissue. Needles of 8 mm in length are used with a pinch-up technique except in obese patients, in whom the standard 12 mm needle should be used. When insulin is being injected without pinch-up into the arms, 6 mm needles are recommended. It is no longer considered necessary to swab the skin with alcohol or to withdraw the skin plunger to check for blood. Care must be taken in thin patients to avoid intramuscular injection as this will result in more rapid absorption of insulin.

Figure 3.6 Usual sites of insulin administration are the outer thighs, buttocks, upper arms and abdomen, and should be rotated within each anatomic area as injection into exactly the same site may cause lipohypertrophy), which may hinder insulin absorption. Insulin absorption may vary from one site to another.

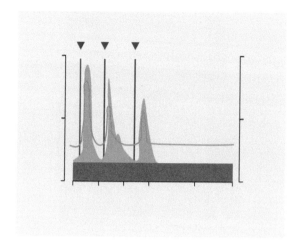

Figure 3.8 Physiologic plasma insulin and glucose profiles: In non-diabetic subjects, basal fasting insulin secretion is very low and suppresses hepatic glucose production, but meal ingestion results in a rapid increase in insulin secretion (shown here). This tight regulation keeps plasma glucose concentrations within a narrow range of about 3.5–7.5 mmol/l (63–135 mg/dl). It is this pattern which exogenous insulin therapy attempts to emulate.

provide very stable insulin concentrations when given in once-daily dosing. In the case of Tresiba, this is achieved as the insulin aggregates into long polymeric chains in the subcutaneous space with slow dissociation to release insulin monomers. In the case of Toujeo, insulin glargine is standardised to 300 u/ml rather than the more usual 100 units/ml, and the increased concentration results in lower solubility and slower absorption into the circulation. Both Toujeo and Tresiba have been shown to be associated with less hypoglycaemia in clinical trials when compared to the first-generation insulin analogues (Figures 3.8–3.11).

DIETARY MANAGEMENT AND PATIENT EDUCATION

There has been little consensus over time on optimal dietary advice for patients with T1DM. General principles have been to maintain a moderate restriction in carbohydrates and a low-fat content in the diet. In the DCCT, only broad dietary advice was provided but it was noted that the regularity of the diet and some adjustment of insulin for carbohydrates were associated with better outcomes. At the same time in Europe, interest was developing

in a more formalised approach to adjustment of insulin for carbohydrates and this approach was developed and refined in Dusseldorf, Germany, as the basis for a five-day residential structured education programme in which patients were taught the basic principles of insulin adjustment based on ratios of insulin to carbohydrate. Audit data from this programme showed very good attainment of HbA$_{1C}$ targets but with less hypoglycaemia than seen for similar levels of glycaemic control in

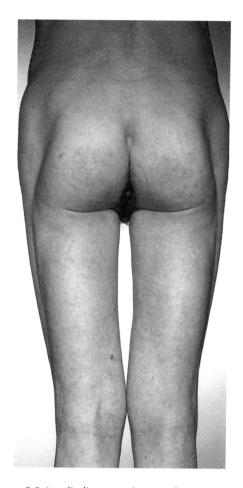

Figure 3.9 Insulin lipoatrophy manifests as depressed areas of skin owing to underlying fat atrophy. This was common before the advent of purified porcine and, more especially, human insulin. Several rare syndromes of lipoatrophy associated with diabetes have been described and are characterized by insulin-resistant diabetes and absence of subcutaneous adipose tissue, either generalized or partial. These syndromes constitute a heterogeneous group, some of which are congenital and others of which are acquired.

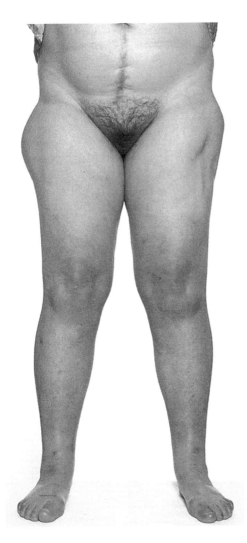

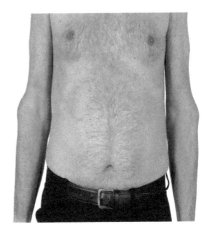

Figure 3.11 This patient has areas of lipohyper-trophy on both elbows. This is a highly unusual site to encounter lipid hypertrophy and a highly unusual site for insulin injection. His glycemic control, as a consequence, was very unstable but improved when he was persuaded to inject elsewhere on a rotational basis.

Figure 3.10 This patient has both insulin lipid hypertrophy and lipoatrophy. The lipid hyper-trophy is seen in the lateral thigh and buttock regions where insulin has been injected. If the same injection site is used over many years, a soft fatty dermal nodule, often of considerable size, develops, possibly owing to the lipogenic action of insulin. Patients should be discouraged from using such sites as variation in insulin absorption may occur, leading to erratic control.

the DCCT. In the UK, the Dusseldorf model was adapted to form the basis of the Dose Adjustment for Normal Eating (DAFNE)-structured education programme, and this and similar programmes have now formed the basis of T1DM self-manage-ment education. DAFNE advocates adjustment of insulin for a 'normal' diet and imposes no specific advice on carbohydrate intake or other dietary measures other than general advice on healthy eating. Participants are taught to adjust mealtime insulin on a meal-by-meal basis using a ratio of insulin to carbohydrate portions (1 portion being 10 g) and to adjust basal insulin replacement according to overall glucose patterns observed over time. In a randomised controlled trial, the DAFNE programme was shown to be associated with improved HbA_{1C} and perceived quality of life, and this has since been confirmed in real-world audit data collected at scale across the UK with additional evidence being observed of a reduc-tion in severe hypoglycaemia and improvement in hypoglycaemia awareness. On the basis of these results, DAFNE and similar-structured education programmes have been made a standard of care for type 1 management in national guidelines and var-ious tools including carbohydrate tables and apps have been developed to support self-management.

GLUCOSE MONITORING

A limiting factor in the management of T1DM has been the need for frequent blood glucose monitor-ing with many patients needing to test glucose more than eight times a day to achieve optimal glucose control. The challenges of performing large num-bers of finger-prick blood tests have meant that many patients found the practice difficult to sus-tain. In recent years, the widespread deployment of subcutaneous continuous glucose monitoring systems has transformed the lives of people with diabetes, reducing the burden of testing and improving outcomes. These systems are based primarily on the use of the glucose oxidase reaction to measure glucose in subcutaneous fluid via a subcutaneous filament. Glucose data are updated every 5 minutes and transmitted to a smartphone or dedicated monitoring device either intermittently using near-field connection technology (described as 'Flash' glucose monitoring) or continuously via a Bluetooth connection.

The use of either intermittently scanned or continuous glucose monitoring has now been endorsed as the standard of care for T1DM patients by NICE in the UK, by the American Diabetes Association and in many other management guidelines. This follows demonstration of efficacy in clinical trials and particularly in large-scale real-world data reviews. Of particular note, the UK ABCD audit of the use of the Abbott Freestyle Libre, the first 'Flash' monitoring system, included data on more than 10,000 people living with diabetes who started using the Freestyle Libre. For patients with more than 7 months of available data, there was a significant reduction in HbA_{1C} from 67.5 mmol/l to 62.3 mmol/l (8.3% to 7.9%) and a more marked reduction among those who had higher HbA_{1C} at entry. In addition, significant reductions were seen in hypoglycaemia frequency and hospital attendance for hypoglycaemia or ketoacidosis.

Continuous glucose sensing technology continues to develop with increasing accuracy, longer duration of individual sensor life and the availability of sensors that do not require calibration by blood glucose measurements. While most systems used in the management of T1DM are based on a subcutaneous filament, a transcutaneous needle-free system (My Sugar Watch) has recently been launched. This device can record glucose for up to 14 hours and may offer an alternative for patients who have had recurrent issues with placement of the more conventional sensors and those where intermittent glucose monitoring to guide insulin titration may be sufficient to support diabetes management.

With the rise in continuous glucose monitoring, a need has arisen for standardised presentation of continuous glucose data, and this has been fulfilled by the development of the ambulatory glucose profile which shows a statistical summary

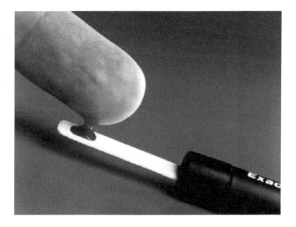

Figure 3.12 Traditional blood glucose self-monitoring based on the glucose oxidase reaction creating an electrical current proportional to its glucose concentration. Frequent self-monitoring has now been superseded by the widespread use of continuous glucose monitoring systems, but is still required to confirm an abnormal glucose and, in some countries, to comply with legal requirements for driving.

of glucose data over a standardised 24 hours alongside data on time in range, with an accepted standard definition of time in range of 3.9–10 mmol/l for this purpose. Continuous glucose data can also be used to estimate HbA_{1C} with the term 'glucose management indicator' being used for this purpose. Where data are available for greater than 60 days, the calculated glucose management indicator is closely correlated to the laboratory HbA_{1C} and is increasingly used as a measure of control in clinical practice (Figures 3.12–3.16).

INSULIN PUMP TREATMENT AND CLOSED-LOOP INSULIN DELIVERY

Insulin pumps were first introduced in the 1980s to enable continuous subcutaneous insulin infusion (CSII), but early experience was variable and was hampered by the limitations of the technology available at the time. A particular issue in early pump experience was an increased risk of diabetic ketoacidosis due to failure of subcutaneous insulin delivery; this is a greater risk for pump users as there is no subcutaneous buffer of insulin to enter the circulation if delivery fails. Through the 1990s, insulin pumps evolved with improvements in microelectronics and started to enter mainstream diabetes care.

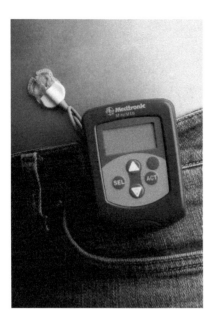

CSII has the advantage over basal bolus insulin delivery by being able to more closely mimic physiological insulin levels and allow for variation in basal insulin delivery rates over the course of the day to match diurnal variations in insulin sensitivity and the effects of exercise. Bolus doses can be precisely matched to carbohydrates and the timing of bolus insulin delivery can be adjusted for different types of meals and to allow for delayed gastric emptying in patients with autonomic dysfunction and gastroparesis.

These advantages have translated into better overall blood glucose control and a reduction in hypoglycaemia burden, including a reduction in severe hypoglycaemia. With the advent of glucose sensor technology, closed-loop insulin pump systems have been developed that modulate insulin delivery based on changes in glucose. While still requiring input of carbohydrate data to optimise mealtime insulin delivery, these systems can

Figure 3.13 The MiniMed continuous glucose monitoring system was the first widely available system to monitor glucose levels in interstitial fluid. In this system, the sensor is inserted under the skin of the anterior abdominal wall and interstitial glucose levels are sensed every 10 seconds and averaged over 5 minutes. The original glucose sensors lasted a maximum of 3 days and required calibration on the basis of four or more capillary glucose readings each day.

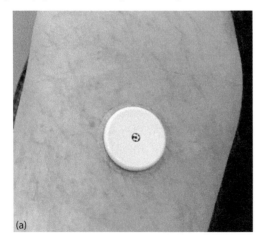

(a)

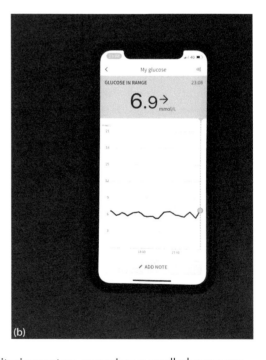

(b)

Figure 3.14 The Freestyle Libre 2 flash glucose monitoring system comprises a small glucose sensor with a subcutaneous filament placed on the arm and measures interstitial fluid glucose for up to 14 days (a). In contrast to earlier continuous glucose monitoring systems, the Libre 2 system does not provide a continuous display of glucose data but blood glucose is measured when desired by 'scanning' the sensor with a reader device or with a smartphone equipped with near-field connectivity (b). The relative simplicity and lower cost of the Libre has allowed for very wide uptake and transformation in monitoring in type 1 diabetes such that the use of continuous monitoring is now accepted as the standard of care for type 1 diabetes in the UK.

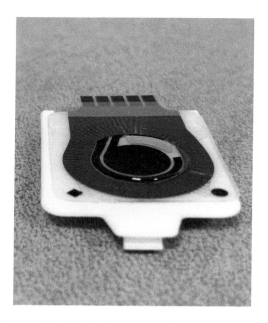

Figure 3.15 The MySugarWatch® glucose sensor system is the first marketed needle free continuous glucose monitor. The sensor comprises a hydrocolloid patch placed over an area of prepared skin on the arm and provides continuous glucose data for up to 14 hours. This may provide a simpler solution for glucose monitoring for those who do not wish to use a sensor on a continuous basis and for intermittent use to support insulin titration in type 2 diabetes.

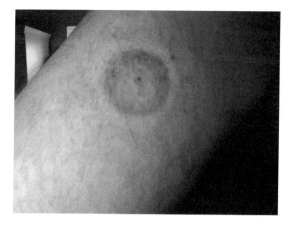

Figure 3.17 With the increased use of wearable technology in type 1 diabetes, there has emerged a small subset of patients who experience significant skin reactions to adhesive used to hold sensors and pump cannulae in place. Here, there is marked erythema at the site of a Freestyle Libre sensor that persisted for more than 48 hours after removal. Although rare, such reactions can limit the use of technology for some individuals.

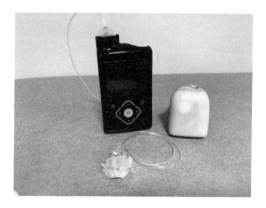

Figure 3.16 Two examples of current insulin pumps; the Medtronic 780 G, a conventional tubed pump, and the Omnipod tubeless insulin delivery system. The Omnipod has a smaller form factor and the infusion site is directly in line with the body of the pump and is controlled by a separate handheld controller. The Medtronic 780 G delivers insulin through a length of tubing and cannula and the controller is integral to the body of the pump.

minimise glucose excursions and enable remarkably tight blood glucose control with very low risks of hypoglycaemia (Figures 3.17–3.19).

PSYCHOLOGICAL ASPECTS OF TYPE 1 DIABETES MANAGEMENT

Despite the advances in medical management that have occurred over recent years, many people with T1DM still struggle to maintain optimal diabetes control and the complexity of management can in itself create a significant psychological burden. There is increasing recognition of the psychological impact of diabetes and a specific concept of 'diabetes distress' has emerged, reflecting feelings of being overwhelmed or failing with diabetes management. Furthermore, a state of 'diabetes burnout' has been identified which can make it hard for an individual to sustain the high level of self-motivation needed for optimal self-management. Incorporating consideration of the psychological impact of diabetes care into routine clinical management is now being recognised as a core element of service provision and consultation

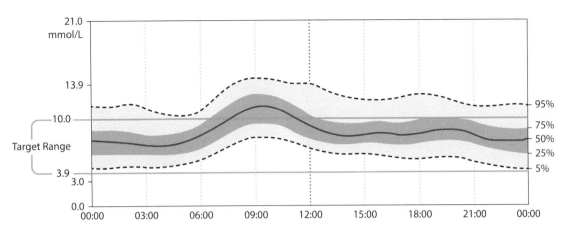

Figure 3.18 The ambulatory glucose profile has been developed as a standard way of summarising data over time from continuous glucose monitoring (CGM) systems and is now used across many platforms. The dark blue line shows the median glucose and this is superimposed on a representation of the interquartile range for glucose. In this case based on continuous data collected over 60 days, there is a pattern of high glucose excursions after breakfast despite otherwise good overall glucose control.

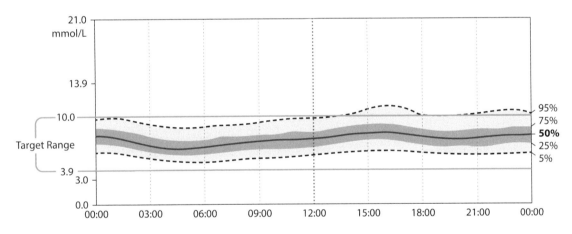

Figure 3.19 With the advent of closed-loop technology, it has proved possible to obtain very consistent blood glucose control with minimal prandial variation and absence of hypoglycaemia as seen in this ambulatory glucose profile trace from a patient using a closed-loop system.

tools that include consideration of diabetes distress and other patient-reported outcome and experience measures have been developed, with evidence that their deployment is associated with improvements in both psychological well-being and glycaemic control. With the ever-growing complexity of diabetes care, the development of effective management pathways to manage the psychological demands of diabetes will be essential to achieve optimal outcomes and help avoid the morbidity that can be associated with suboptimally managed T1DM (Figure 3.20).

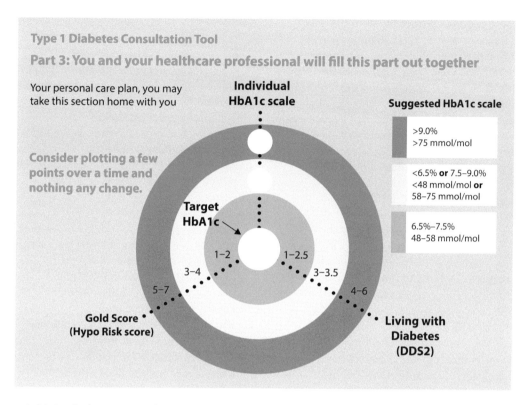

Figure 3.20 With the increased recognition of the impact of psychological factors in diabetes, care tools have been advised to provide simple feedback on a patient's control across various dimensions of care and experience. This type 1 diabetes consultation tool was devised by the SE London Health Innovation Network and presents data on hypoglycaemia awareness, diabetes distress and glycaemic control on a 'dart board' diagram. Use of the tool has been shown to be associated with improved patient satisfaction in consultation and an improvement in distress and HbA$_{1c}$ on follow up.

(From Todd PJ, Edwards F, Spratling L, et al. Evaluating the relationships of hypoglycaemia and HbA$_{1c}$ with screening-detected diabetes distress in type 1 diabetes. Endocrinol Diab Metab. 2018; 1:e3. https://doi.org/10.1002/edm2.3.)

BIBLIOGRAPHY

Bode BW, Steed RD, Davidson PC. Reduction in severe hypoglycemia with long-term continuous subcutaneous insulin infusion in type I diabetes. Diabetes Care. 1996; 19(4): 324–7. doi: 10.2337/diacare.19.4.324

Da Silva J, et al. Real-world performance of the MiniMed™ 780G system: First report of outcomes from 4120 users. Diabetes Technol Ther. 2021. doi: 10.1089/dia.2021.0203

DAFNE study group. Training in flexible, intensive insulin management to enable dietary freedom in people with type 1 diabetes: Dose adjustment for normal eating (DAFNE) randomised controlled trial. BMJ 2002; 325. doi: https://doi.org/10.1136/bmj.325.7367.746

DeVries JH, Snoek FJ, Heine RJ. Persistent poor glycaemic control in adult type 1 diabetes. A closer look at the problem. Diabetic Med. 2004; 21: 1263–8

Hopkins D, Lawrence I, Mansell P, et al. Improved biomedical and psychological outcomes 1 year after structured education in flexible insulin therapy for people with type 1 diabetes: The U.K. DAFNE experience. Diabetes Care. 2012 Aug; 35(8):1638–42. doi: 10.2337/dc11-1579

Khan A, Choudhary P. Investigating the association between diabetes distress and self-management behaviors. J Diabetes Sci Technol. 2018 Nov; 12(6): 1116–24. doi: 10.1177/1932296818789721

Leelarathna L, Little SA, Walkinshaw E, et al. Restoration of self-awareness of hypoglycemia in adults with long-standing type 1 diabetes: Hyperinsulinemic-hypoglycemic clamp substudy results from the HypoCOMPaSS trial. Diabetes Care. 2013 Dec; 36(12): 4063–70. doi: 10.2337/dc13-1004

Mühlhauser I, Jörgens V, Berger M, et al. Bicentric evaluation of a teaching and treatment programme for type 1 (insulin-dependent) diabetic patients: Improvement of metabolic control and other measures of diabetes care for up to 22 months. Diabetologia. 1983 Dec; 25(6): 470–6. doi: 10.1007/BF00284453

Nathan DM. Realising the long-term promise of insulin therapy: The DCCT/EDIC study. Diabetologia. 2021; 64: 1049–58. https://doi.org/10.1007/s00125-021-05397-4

National Institute for Health and Care Excellence. Type 1 diabetes in adults: diagnosis and management. Evidence reviews for long acting insulins in type 1 diabetes. Published online https://www.nice.org.uk/guidance/ng17/evidence/a-longacting-insulins-in-type-1-diabetes-pdf-9196139918

NHS Digital. National Diabetes Audit 2020–21, England & Wales. Published online 16th June 2022 at https://files.digital.nhs.uk/56/9D4E2F/NDA%202020-21%20Type%201%20Diabetes%20Report.pdf

Russell-Jones D, Gall MA, Niemeyer M, et al. Insulin degludec results in lower rates of nocturnal hypoglycaemia and fasting plasma glucose vs. insulin glargine: A meta-analysis of seven clinical trials. Nutr Metab Cardiovasc Dis. 2015 Oct; 25(10): 898–905. doi: 10.1016/j.numecd.2015.06.005

The Diabetes Control and Complications Trial Research Group. Progression of long-term complications in insulin-dependent diabetes mellitus. N Engl J Med 1993; 329: 977–86. doi: 10.1056/NEJM199309303291401

4

Treatment of type 2 diabetes mellitus

In the early years of insulin management of diabetes, it was recognised that there was a subset of patients who had less severe metabolic derangement and who could be managed by dietary measures without insulin, particularly with weight loss. These individuals generally developed diabetes at an older age and, thus, the term 'maturity onset diabetes' became prevalent. Studies performed in the late 1940s and early 1950s using insulin bioassays showed that these individuals had preserved circulating insulin, albeit at a lower level than in healthy control subjects. Out of this work, the concept emerged that this type of diabetes was due to insulin resistance and a relevant impairment in insulin secretion in contrast to the absolute insulin deficiency of the classical syndrome of what we now consider as type 1 diabetes mellitus (T1DM). This syndrome was variously described as 'maturity onset diabetes' and 'non-insulin dependent diabetes' until standardised terminology was adopted following a World Health Organization (WHO) consensus report in 1999, when the current classifications of T1DM and type 2 diabetes mellitus (T2DM) were adopted.

Historically, what we now call T2DM was considered to be a less-severe form of diabetes than T1DM on the basis that acute metabolic decompensation was rare. Many patients were treated only on the basis of avoiding osmotic symptoms associated with marked hyperglycaemia. However, epidemiological data emerged to show that far from being a mild disease, T2DM was associated with significant morbidity and mortality and with a similar range of diabetes complications to those seen in T1DM.

This led to studies being carried out to assess the impact of glucose control on diabetes complications and conclusive evidence of this came with the publication of the United Kingdom Prospective Diabetes Study (UKPDS) study in 1998. This large, long-term intervention study recruited a cohort of more than 5000 people with T2DM from the point of diagnosis with randomisation to standard control based on symptomatic management of diabetes versus a regime of 'tight blood glucose control' based on achieving near normal glucose levels. In a substudy, 1148 patients were also randomised into 'tight' versus standard blood pressure control groups. Given the limitations of glucose medication at the time of onset of the study, management was based first on sulphonylurea for the majority of patients and on metformin for a subset of those who were overweight at recruitment.

After a median of 10 years of follow-up, there was a 0.9% difference in HbA_{1C} between the two groups (7.0% for the intensive arm and 7.9% for the conventional arm). This difference was associated with significantly lower rates of development and progression of microvascular disease in the intensive management arm with a risk reduction of microvascular endpoints of 25% and a non-significant trend to lower cardiovascular events. In those starting with metformin as a first-line treatment, the overall risk reduction was greater. In the blood pressure substudy, a difference in attained BP of 12/7 mmHg (142/82 mmHg *versus* 154/87 mmHg over a median of 8.4 years) achieved with the use of ACE inhibitors or beta blockers reduced the risk of both microvascular and macrovascular disease.

Following the completion of the randomised UKPDS study, participants continued to be followed for a further 10 years. During this time, the difference in blood glucose control between the two arms was lost with intensification of management in the control subjects. However, the separation between the two groups in outcomes persisted

DOI: 10.1201/9781003342700-4

with a 24% reduction in microvascular endpoints. In addition, significant relative risk reductions emerged for myocardial infarction (15%) and all-cause mortality (12%). These results indicated a 'legacy effect' of early, tight blood glucose control that persisted for many years. A similar legacy effect was also seen in other, smaller outcome studies, but, in contrast, studies of intensification of control later in the course of diabetes have shown less benefit and, in one case, an increase in cardiovascular events.

These results had a profound impact on the development of T2DM management in the early years of the 20th century, aided by the appearance of an extended range of drugs for the management of T2DM. Current guidelines now recommend aiming for near normoglycaemia following diagnosis, with an ideal target HbA_{1C} of 48 mmol/mol (6.5%) for patients on drugs with a low risk of hypoglycaemia and of 53 mmol/mol (7.0%) for those on other agents.

DIETARY TREATMENT FOR T2DM

Although the majority of people with T2DM will begin pharmacotherapy early after the diagnosis of diabetes, diet remains a pivotal aspect of management. Over 80% of people with T2DM are overweight or obese at diagnosis, and targeting weight loss should be a key aspect of dietary management. In a recent review of the literature, weight loss of approximately 5% of body weight was required to achieve a significant effect on blood glucose control and this was associated with a 7 mmol/mol fall in HbA_{1C} in patients with established diabetes and up to 13 mmol/mol reduction in those with newly diagnosed diabetes. Furthermore, patients who succeeded with weight loss were more likely to sustain target HbA_{1C} over a longer period.

Simple initial advice for calorie restriction and avoidance of sweet foods and drinks can lead to symptomatic improvement and a reduction in blood glucose levels before any reductions in body weight are detectable, but ongoing support and a strategic approach to supporting weight management are required for effective intervention. There remains little consensus over dietary constituency other than for a need for caloric restriction. Moderate carbohydrate restriction and an overall reduction in fat (particularly saturates) is generally recommended.

There is increased interest in more marked dietary measures aiming at achieving higher levels of weight loss and remission of diabetes altogether in the early years after diagnosis. This was the approach of the DIRECT study which used an 800 kCal meal-replacement programme followed by a gradual reintroduction of a normal diet, with the aim of achieving and sustaining a 15 kg weight loss. In an initial cluster randomised study of the intervention, a mean weight reduction of 10 kg was observed and 46% of participants achieved remission of diabetes, with greater rates of remission among those with the greatest achieved weight loss.

In most clinical services, dietary self-management guidance is provided as part of a structured education programme such as the Diabetes Education and Self -Management for Ongoing and Newly Diagnosed diabetes (DESMOND) programme which aims to provide general advice on living with diabetes and support the development of self-efficacy. In randomised studies, this and similar interventions were shown to be associated with greater weight loss and greater understanding of diabetes, but in contrast to programmes in T1DM, observed impact on HbA_{1C} has been limited, reflecting the difficulty sustaining control in T2DM without achieving significant weight loss or the introduction of pharmacotherapy.

DRUG TREATMENT FOR T2DM

Oral alternatives to insulin for the management of T2DM first emerged with the introduction of sulphonylureas and metformin in the 1950s. These remained the mainstay of diabetes management until the 1990s when rapid advances in the understanding of T2DM led to the appearance of a range of new medications with novel mechanisms of action. The past 20 years have seen progressive improvement in the pharamacotherapy of T2DM, incorporating learning from large scale clinical trials of these newer agents (Figure 4.1).

SULPHONYLUREAS

The first commercially available sulphonylurea was launched in 1956, and this class of drugs became the mainstay of diabetes treatment until the start of the 21st century. Sulphonylureas stimulate insulin secretion from the beta cell (β-cell) by binding to and inducing closure of ATP-sensitive potassium channels that play a key role in the regulation of insulin secretion. As a result of their mechanism of action, sulphonylureas are only effective in patients with preserved insulin secretion and,

Drug class	Primary mechanism of action	Year first introduced
Insulin	Direct stimulation of glucose uptake in cells	1923
Sulphonylureas	Enhance insulin secretion acting via KATP channel closure	1955
Biguanides	Reduce hepatic glucose output and increase insulin sensitivity	1957
α–glucosidase inhibitor	Prevent breakdown of oligosaccharides in small intestine and thus reduce absorption of glucose	1990
Meglitinides	Enhance insulin secretion acting via KATP channel closure	1994
Thiazolidinediones	Activate transcription factor PPARγ increasing expression of multiple insulin signaling proteins	1995
GLP-1 receptor agonists	Stimulate insulin secretion, reduce gastric emptying and promote satiety acting through GLP-1 receptor	2005
DPP IV inhibitors	Increase circulating concentration of native GLP-1 by inhibition of degradation	2006
SGLT-2 Inhibitors	Promote glycosuria through inhibition of proximal tubule glucose reabsorption	2013
GLP-1/GIP dual agonists	As GLP-1 RA with additional effects at GIP receptor	2022

Figure 4.1 A timeline of the introduction of drugs for the treatment of type 2 diabetes.

thus, their effect declines over time as progressive β-cell failure is a characteristic of T2DM. As they stimulate insulin secretion across a wide range of glucose levels, they carry some risk of hypoglycaemia, particularly in situations where the drug and active metabolites may accumulate, such as in renal failure. There has been a gradual evolution of sulphonylureas with older agents (chlorpropamide and glibenclamide) having a long duration of action and predominant renal excretion, resulting in a greater hypoglycaemia risk. Newer agents such as glimepiride and gliclazide are predominatly metabolised in the liver and are associated with less hypoglycaemia.

While there is a strong evidence base for the efficacy of the sulphonylureas (which were a first-line treatment for the majority of patients in the UKPDS), their use is declining due to their association with weight gain and hypoglycaemia and the lack of specific cardiovascular benefits in comparison to newer agents.

BIGUANIDES (METFORMIN)

The first biguanide phenformin entered clinical use in 1958, but was later withdrawn due to an association with lactic acidosis, a potentially lethal acute metabolic derangement. A second biguanide, metformin, remained available in Europe, but was only approved in the US in 1994. Metformin lowers plasma glucose primarily by inhibiting hepatic glucose production and increasing the sensitivity of peripheral tissue to insulin. It does not usually cause hypoglycaemia but, as it is renally excreted, it can accumulate and its use is relatively contraindicated in patients with renal and hepatic impairment due to an associated risk of lactic acidosis. It is weight neutral and on this basis was used as a first-line treatment in a subgroup of overweight patients in the UKPDS study. The overall results in terms of risk reduction in this group were slightly better than for those starting with sulphonylurea and, as a result, metformin has become a mainstay of diabetes management, remaining as the first-line oral agent for the majority of patients.

Gastrointestinal side-effects are common, including bloating, dyspepsia and altered taste. These effects are dose dependent and can generally be minimized by gradual dose titration. To minimize the occurrence of side-effects, patients should start on a low dose. Weight gain is usually not a problem with metformin, possibly because it has a slight anorectic effect.

α-GLUCOSIDASE INHIBITORS

These drugs, which include acarbose (Glucobay®, Bayer) were introduced in the mid-1990s and have been widely used as a first-line treatment in some countries. They delay the absorption of complex carbohydrates from the gastrointestinal tract and are of value in controlling postprandial hyperglycaemia; however, their blood glucose lowering effect is modest and lower than those of metformin or the sulphonylureas, and the side-effects of flatulence and diarrhoea often limit their tolerability. As a result, their use has declined with the emergence of newer agents.

MEGLITINIDES

This class of agents comprises two drugs, repaglinide and nateglinide. They were first introduced in the late 1990s and are similar in their action to sulphonylureas, acting via closure of K-ATP channels in the β-cells, although their receptor-binding characteristics are different. Compared to sulphonylureas, their effect on insulin is short lived and is dependent on the concentration of glucose. Thus, taken before meals, they restore towards normal the impaired insulin response to meals seen in T2DM, with a lower overall risk of hypoglycaemia than seen with sulphonylureas. However, as a result of their short duration of action, they need to be taken with each meal to be effective. While they offer an alternative to sulphonylureas, for some patients, their use has been limited and has declined with the arrival of newer agents.

THIAZOLINEIDIONES (GLITAZONES)

These drugs work by activating the nuclear receptor peroxisome proliferator-activated receptor-gamma (PPARγ), which is found predominantly in adipose tissue, but also in skeletal muscle and liver. This leads to the upregulation of expression of several proteins in the insulin signalling pathway, effectively sensitizing target tissues to insulin and resulting in a reduction of hepatic glucose production and an increase in peripheral glucose uptake. Thiazolidinediones act to increase fatty-acid uptake into adipocytes, thus, lowering triglyceride and non-esterified fatty-acid levels which also contribute to the favourable effects of the drugs on glucose metabolism outlined previously. These agents can be very effective at lowering glucose in patients with marked insulin resistance and, at the time of their initial launch, there was considerable interest in their potential to influence cardiovascular outcomes due to an apparently favourable effect on lipids and other potential risk markers.

However, the promise of these agents was not borne out in clinical practice. The first agent to reach market, Troglitazone, was found to have significant hepatoxicity in some users and was rapidly withdrawn. Two other agents, Rosiglitazone and Pioglitazone, were widely used in the early 2000s, but Rosiglitazone was later withdrawn from the market after concerns of a possible data signal of increased cardiovascular mortality. Pioglitazone remains available, but its use has declined. While an effective drug for lowering blood glucose, its use is associated with weight gain and fluid retention, which can exacerbate heart failure in some patients. A study designed to determine if pioglitazone had cardiovascular benefit over other available drugs (PROACTIVE) was inconclusive, with no benefit seen in the prespecified composite primary endpoint, though some secondary endpoint data did suggest possible benefits.

INCRETIN-BASED TREATMENTS

The first major advance in treatment of T2DM in the 21st century was the launch of incretin-based therapies, firstly with the glucagon-like peptide-1 (GLP-1) agonist drug exenatide in 2005 and the first dipeptidyl peptidase-4 (DPP-IV) inhibitor sitagliptin in 2006. The development of these drugs resulted from the identification of incretins, gut-derived peptides that enhance glucose-mediated insulin secretion and have a range of additional effects, notably slowing of gastric emptying that enhances postprandial glucose control. The two major incretins are GLP-1 and gastric inhibitory polypeptide (GIP). GLP-1 was the initial target of pharmacological research, as GLP-1 levels are low in T2DM and early studies demonstrated that GLP-1 infusion was effective at stimulating insulin secretion and lowering glucose. However, native human GLP-1 has a plasma half-life of less than 5 minutes, limiting its therapeutic potential and leading to the need to develop stable agonists. Two principal groups of injectable GLP-1 agonist drugs have now been developed based on Exendin, a more stable lizard-derived GLP-1-like molecule (e.g. exenatide and lixisenatide) and based on modification of the sequence of human GLP-1 (e.g. liraglutide, semaglutide and dulaglutide) to enhance protein-binding in the circulation from degradation.

A second therapeutic approach has been the development of inhibitors of DPP-IV, a ubiquitous protease enzyme that is primarily responsible for the degradation of circulating native GLP-1. A series of potent DPP-IV inhibitors have now been developed which indirectly stimulate insulin secretion by potentiating the levels of circulating GLP-1.

The GLP-1 agonists are potent glucose-lowering agents that also have a significant impact on weight; indeed, several agents in the class are now licensed for the treatment of obesity outside of the context of diabetes management. As their primary glucose-lowering effect is through stimulation of insulin secretion, they rely on the presence of residual β-cell function and become less effective late in the course of diabetes when β-cell failure has become prominent. In contrast to sulphonylureas, their effect on insulin secretion is glucose dependent and attenuated at low glucose concentrations. As a result, they are associated with a low risk of hypoglycaemia compared to sulphonyl-ureas and insulin. While the original GLP-1 drugs required once or twice daily administration, second generation GLP-1 agonists (semaglutide, dulaglutide and extended release exenatide) have been developed that allow the convenience of once daily administration, reducing the treatment burden associated with injectable treatments.

The DPP-IV inhibitors are less potent than GLP-1 agonists, reflecting the fact that they elevate circulating GLP-1 levels to high physiological concentrations compared to the supraphysiological effect of the agonist drugs. They are effective at lowering blood glucose and carry a lower risk of hypoglycaemia than sulphonylureas, but do not have any significant effect on weight. They are increasingly used in place of sulphonylureas in the oral treatment of T2DM.

A new development in the incretin field is the launch of the first dual incretin agonist, tirzepatide, which entered clinical practice in the US in late 2022. Tirzepatide has actions at both the GLP-1 and GIP receptor and, in clinical trials, was shown to have very high potency in glucose lowering and particularly in supporting weight loss. It is likely to assume a major role in the management of T2DM, particularly in obese subjects (Figure 4.2).

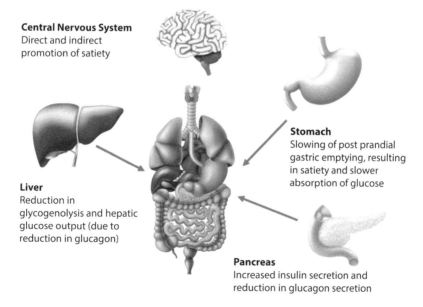

Central Nervous System
Direct and indirect promotion of satiety

Stomach
Slowing of post prandial gastric emptying, resulting in satiety and slower absorption of glucose

Liver
Reduction in glycogenolysis and hepatic glucose output (due to reduction in glucagon)

Pancreas
Increased insulin secretion and reduction in glucagon secretion

Figure 4.2 Actions of GLP-1 receptor agonists relevant to glucose homeostasis. The primary action of GLP-1 is to promote glucose-dependent insulin secretion in pancreatic β-cells. In addition, GLP-1 RA treatment is associated with a slowing of gastric emptying and a reduction in glucagon secretion from pancreatic alpha cells. This results in a reduction in peak postprandial glucose absorption and hepatic glucose output, which, together with the increase in insulin secretion, leads to a reduction in post-prandial hyperglycaemia. In addition to the effect on gastric emptying, GLP-1 RA has direct but as yet not fully elucidated effects on appetite control in the central nervous system and the promotion of satiety is a major contributor to the weight loss observed following GLP-1 RA treatment.

SGLT-2 INHIBITORS

The first SGLT-2 (Sodium-Glucose Co-transporter) inhibitor entered clinical practice at the end of 2013 and, since then, this class of drugs has become a mainstay of T2DM treatment, with three agents (canagliflozin, dapagliflozin and empagliflozin) in widespread use. The principle behind their action is that glucose is filtered freely in the glomerulus of the kidney, but most of the filtered glucose is reabsorbed from the renal tubular system by sodium-glucose co-transporters. There are two principal types of transporter in the kidney—SGLT-1 and SGLT-2—with the latter present primarily in the proximal tubule and being responsible for reabsorption of approximately 90% of the filtered glucose. Inhibition of SGLT-2 results in significant renal glucose excretion with a concomitant reduction on blood glucose and potential for weight loss. In clinical trials, SGLT-2 inhibitors were found to be highly effective at lowering blood glucose and to be generally weight tolerant. In addition, they were shown to have multiple additional effects of potential benefit, including lowering blood pressure and reducing proteinuria in patients with established diabetic kidney disease. There are some potential adverse effects; the high urinary glucose load predisposes to genito-urinary infection, particularly genital candidiasis, and this can be a limiting factor for some patients. In addition, in patients with significant insulin deficiency, SGLT-2 treatment can predispose to the development of ketoacidosis and a specific phenomenon of ketoacidosis occurring without marked elevation of glucose (euglycaemic ketoacidosis). For this reason, ketone monitoring should be considered for patients who are also on insulin treatment and SGLT-2 inhibitors should be stopped during intercurrent illness that may predispose to metabolic decompensation (Figure 4.3).

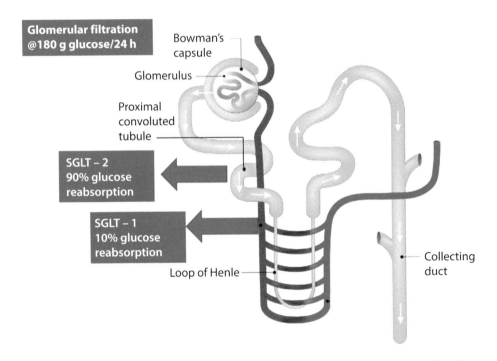

Figure 4.3 Role of SGLT-1 and -2 in renal glucose handling. Glucose is filtered freely in the glomerulus but in health is completely reabsorbed, resulting in minimal renal glucose loss. Reabsorption is mediated in conjunction with reabsorption of sodium by sodium glucose co-transporters (SGLTs) with around 90% of the reabsorption being mediated by SGLT-2 in the proximal tubule. The remaining 10% is then reabsorbed more distally in the tubule by the SGLT-1-mediated transport. In healthy individuals, about 160–180 g of glucose are filtered over a 24 h period. With SGLT-2 inhibition, there is a marked reduction of glucose reabsorption, resulting in about 60–80 g of glucose excretion per day.

INSULIN

If glycaemic control is not sustained despite optimal oral drug treatment or GLP-1 agonist treatment, insulin therapy may be indicated. Insulin is the only effective therapy in T2DM once significant β-cell failure has supervened. Oral agents fail to lower blood glucose levels adequately once the β-cell reserve falls below about 15% of normal.

Approximately half of all T2DM will require insulin therapy because of a progressive decline in β-cell function. Insulin therapy may be associated with an increase in weight and increased risk of hypoglycaemia compared to other treatment regimes, and specific dietary management reinforcement is needed to minimize weight gain.

There are many ways of giving insulin to patients with T2DM and there is no universal consensus on the best way of delivering insulin. There is, however, growing evidence for an approach that starts with once daily long-acting insulin with later introduction of a rapid-acting mealtime insulin, if required. There is also evidence that longer-acting insulin analogues (e.g. Tresiba [insulin degludec] and Toujeo [insulin glargine 300 units/ml]) are associated with a lower risk of hypoglycaemia and a greater likelihood of achieving glucose-control targets without hypoglycaemia.

There is evidence that using a GLP-1 agonist in combination with basal insulin replacement can be more effective than using basal insulin alone, and two preparations combining a basal insulin analogue and a GLP-1 agonist (Xultophy, comprising degludec and liraglutide and Suliqua, comprising lixisenatide and glargine), have now entered clinical practice and have been shown to provide excellent glucose control with less weight gain and hypoglycaemia, reflecting lower overall insulin dose requirements than for insulin-only regimes.

CARDIOVASCULAR OUTCOME STUDIES

A major change in diabetes management has been the recognition that some of the newer agents have advantages in terms of cardiovascular outcomes and reduction in mortality that are independent of their effects on lowering blood glucose. Following concerns about the safety of rosiglitazone, cardiovascular outcome studies were mandated by the US Food and Drug Administration for approval of all new glucose-lowering medications, and this led to the development of very large-scale outcome studies which were designed to show non-inferiority over comparator in cardiovascular safety parameters.

The first of these to report positively was EMPA-REG, a study of empagliflozin, followed by the Liraglutide Effect and Action in Diabetes: Evaluation of Cardiovascular Outcome Results (LEADER) study of the cardiovascular safety of liraglutide. In both studies, significant benefits were seen in terms of a reduction in a composite cardiovascular endpoint. Since then, additional studies have shown evidence of benefit for other GLP-1 receptor agonists (dulaglutide and semaglutide) and other SGLT-2 inhibitors (dapagliflozin and canagliflozin). The effects observed have been variable between studies, reflecting differences in design but, overall, show clear benefits of these newer classes of agents over earlier diabetes treatments. Additional benefits have been seen with SGLT-2 inhibitors in relation to heart failure and progression of proteinuria in diabetic nephropathy and have led to these agents being used earlier in the treatment pathway for T2DM, particularly in patients with pre-existing cardiovascular disease and high overall cardiovascular risk.

TREATMENT STRATEGIES AND GUIDELINES

The wealth of new information that has appeared over recent years has led to a comprehensive review of guidance for the management of T2DM, with particular emphasis on considering an individual's cardiovascular risk and requirements for weight management in choosing initial and subsequent drugs.

Metformin remains the first-line treatment for the majority of patients in whom it is tolerated and in the absence of any contraindications (primarily in relation to renal function). However, for those with high cardiovascular risk, current guidance now recommends the addition of an SGLT-2 inhibitor, either simultaneously as joint first-line treatment or immediately after starting metformin. For obese patients, consideration may be given to early use of GLP-1 agonists (which are now also licenced in the management of prediabetic hyperglycaemia). For those with no specific reason to use either of these agents, then second-line treatment is at individual discretion with a choice of any of the established agents. For many, acquisition cost remains a significant factor in the choice of drug, as the newer agents are significantly more expensive than older diabetes treatments; in the UK GLP-1 agonists remain relatively late in the NICE treatment recommendations compared to other agents, reflecting their high cost.

All current guidelines place a strong emphasis on determining an individual glycaemic target based on factors including age and duration of diabetes and balancing the benefits of tight glycaemic control with risks associated with hypoglycaemia, particularly in the elderly. While there is strong evidence that early intensive management reduces morbidity, the impact of diabetes is related to age at diagnosis with risks of complications being high in those diagnosed at a young age while those diagnosed in their 70s and older have a much lower risk. Hence, an ideal target HbA$_{1C}$ of under 48 or 53 mmol/mol (6.5–7%) may

be set for a young person with new onset T2DM, whereas a target of 64 mmol/mol (8%) may be acceptable at an older age. Once set, it is important that treatment is promptly escalated when control is sustained above target, as real-world data analyses have shown that there is a significant issue with treatment inertia and individual patients often have poor control for many years before treatment is escalated.

Furthermore, treatment of hyperglycaemia in T2DM should be considered as only one aspect of management. T2DM is a multifaceted syndrome with strong associations with hypertension, hyperlipidaemia and cardiovascular disease, and a comprehensive approach to managing these other risk factors is essential to optimise outcomes. The importance of effective self-management should also be given due consideration, as treatment of these various risk factors can carry a significant emotional burden which needs to be addressed to help a person achieve good physical and psychological health despite living with a long-term condition (Figures 4.4 and 4.5).

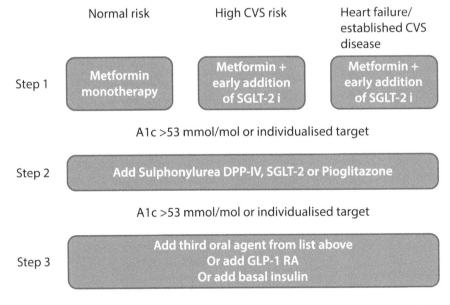

Figure 4.4 A simplified treatment algorithm for management of type 2 diabetes, based on the ADA/EASD and NICE 2022 guidance. Treatment should be aimed at maintaining a HbA$_{1C}$ target of <53 mmol/mol (7.0%) or to an individualised target based on a holistic assessment of the individual. A specific evaluation of cardiovascular risk and the presence or absence of heart failure or other cardiovascular disease should be made to guide treatment.

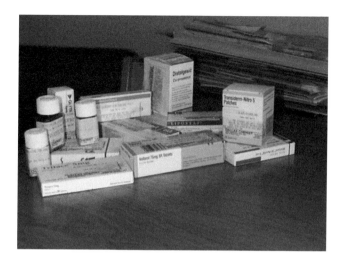

Figure 4.5 The management of type 2 diabetes often results in extensive polypharmacy, which creates particular challenges in concordance and can create a significant burden for those living with diabetes. Consideration of the psychological burden and support in self-efficacy are important aspects of successful management.

BIBLIOGRAPHY

Bornstein J, Lawrence RD. Plasma insulin in human diabetes mellitus. Br Med J. 1951 Dec 29; 2(4747): 1541–4. doi: 10.1136/bmj.2.4747.1541

Davies MJ, Aroda VR, Collins BS, Gabbay RA, Green J, Maruthur NM, Rosas SE, Del Prato S, Mathieu C, Mingrone G, Rossing P, Tankova T, Tsapas A, Buse JB. Management of hypergly-cemia in type 2 diabetes, 2022. A consensus report by the American Diabetes Association (ADA) and the European Association for the Study of Diabetes (EASD). Diabetes Care. 2022 Nov 1; 45(11): 2753–86. doi: 10.2337/dci22-0034

Davies MJ, Heller S, Skinner TC, et al. Effectiveness of the diabetes education and self management for ongoing and newly diagnosed (DESMOND) programme for people with newly diagnosed type 2 diabetes: Cluster randomised controlled trial. BMJ. 2008 Mar 1; 336(7642): 491–5. doi: 10.1136/bmj.39474.922025.BE

Diabetes UK 2018 Nutrition Working Group. Evidence based nutrition guidelines for the prevention and management of diabetes. Published online March 2018 at https://diabetes-resources-production.s3.eu-west-1.amazonaws.com/resources-s3/2018-03/1373_Nutrition%20guidelines_0.pdf

Evans M, Morgan AR, Whyte MB, Hanif W, Bain SC, Kalra PA, Davies S, Dashora U, Yousef Z, Patel DC, Strain WD. New therapeutic horizons in chronic kidney disease: The role of SGLT2 inhibitors in clinical practice. Drugs. 2022 Feb; 82(2): 97–108. doi: 10.1007/s40265-021-01655-2

Holman RR, Farmer AJ, Davies MJ, Levy JC, Darbyshire JL, Keenan JF, Paul SK; 4-T Study Group. Three-year efficacy of complex insulin regimens in type 2 diabetes. N Engl J Med. 2009 Oct 29; 361(18): 1736–47. doi: 10.1056/NEJMoa0905479

Karagiannis T, Avgerinos I, Liakos A, et al. Management of type 2 diabetes with the dual GIP/GLP-1 receptor agonist tirzepa-tide: A systematic review and meta-analysis. Diabetologia. 2022 Aug; 65(8): 1251–61. doi: 10.1007/s00125-022-05715-4

Lean ME, Leslie WS, Barnes AC, et al. Primary care-led weight management for remis-sion of type 2 diabetes (DiRECT): An open-label, cluster-randomised trial. Lancet. 2018 Feb 10; 391(10120): 541–51. doi: 10.1016/S0140-6736(17)33102-1

Marso SP, Daniels GH, Brown-Frandsen K, Kristensen P, Mann JF, Nauck MA, Nissen SE, Pocock S, Poulter NR, Ravn LS, Steinberg WM, Stockner M, Zinman B, Bergenstal RM, Buse JB; LEADER Steering Committee; LEADER Trial Investigators. Liraglutide and cardiovascular outcomes in type 2 diabetes. N Engl J Med. 2016 Jul 28; 375(4): 311–22. doi: 10.1056/NEJMoa1603827

Nauck MA, Quast DR, Wefers J, Meier JJ. GLP-1 receptor agonists in the treatment of type 2 diabetes - state-of-the-art. Mol Metab. 2021 Apr; 46: 101102. doi: 10.1016/j.molmet.2020.101102

Sheahan KH, Wahlberg EA, Gilbert MP. An overview of GLP-1 agonists and recent cardiovascular outcomes trials. Postgrad Med J. 2020 Mar; 96(1133): 156–61. doi: 10.1136/postgradmedj-2019-137186

Turner RC. The U.K. Prospective diabetes study. A review. Diabetes Care. 1998 Dec; 21(Suppl 3): C35–8. doi: 10.2337/diacare.21.3.c35

Zinman B, Wanner C, Lachin JM, Fitchett D, Bluhmki E, Hantel S, Mattheus M, Devins T, Johansen OE, Woerle HJ, Broedl UC, Inzucchi SE; EMPA-REG OUTCOME Investigators. Empagliflozin, cardiovascular outcomes, and mortality in type 2 diabetes. N Engl J Med. 2015 Nov 26; 373(22): 2117–28. doi: 10.1056/NEJMoa1504720

5

Treatment of children and adolescents with diabetes

TYPE 1 DIABETES

The importance of effective strategies for the treatment of diabetes in children and adolescents is accentuated by the knowledge that time-trend data, for countries where it is available, have demonstrated a clear increase in incidence of type 1 diabetes mellitus (T1DM) in these age groups. Such an increase suggests changes in environmental factors, with the larger increase in children <5 years of age, in early life.

Treatment strategies must incorporate knowledge of developmental milestones and the behavioural, physiological, psychological and social factors that operate in this age group and impact so strongly on any chronic disease management programme in children. Emotional problems are common and some studies have suggested that the onset of diabetes is associated with adjustment disorders, which seemed to confer an increased risk of psychiatric problems later in life. A recent prospective study of adolescents with T1DM from Australia documented the exhibition of a broad range of psychological morbidity 10 years after disease onset, with females and adolescents with pre-existing psychological problems being at particular risk.

The management of diabetes in young people needs a comprehensive multidisciplinary approach comprising the paediatrician, specialist nurse, dietitian and psychologist, with provision for progressive transition to adult care, usually starting at the age of 13 years. Close liaison with schools is essential to ensure that appropriate adjustments are in place to enable a pupil to manage diabetes effectively and avoid any stigma related to having to take diabetes treatment at school. Historically, some children with diabetes have been excluded from some sports at school, but the current philosophy of management is to normalise diabetes in everyday activities and to avoid any restrictions.

In recent years, there has been increased emphasis on early optimization of blood glucose control, provided this can be achieved without problematic hypoglycaemia. As a result, there has been a gradual shift away from pre-mixed insulin regimes (which were often used in paediatric practice in the interest of simplicity) to basal bolus insulin regimes and insulin pump treatment. In the UK, insulin pump treatment is now recommended as a primary option for children under the age of 12 years and for older children where there is sustained poor glucose control or HbA_{1C} >72 mmol/mol (8.5%). Total daily insulin requirements in children with T1DM are around 0.8 units/kg/24 hours, increasing to 1.0–1.5 units/kg/24 hours in mid-puberty.

The use of continuous glucose monitoring has now become the standard of care for T1DM in children and young people and has the additional advantage in minors that most systems now have the facility for remote monitoring, allowing a parent to maintain sight of a child's blood glucose levels when at school.

TYPE 2 DIABETES IN CHILDREN AND YOUNG PEOPLE

Early onset type 2 diabetes mellitus (T2DM) appearing in children and adolescents started to emerge about 30 years ago as a rare phenomenon. Since then, the prevalence of this condition

DOI: 10.1201/9781003342700-5

has increased progressively, mirroring a rise in childhood obesity in the developed world. In the UK, estimates based on data from 2018 suggested that there were about 800 children with a diagnosis of T2DM and most paediatric diabetes services will now cater to several children with this condition. Children with T2DM are more likely to come from socially deprived family backgrounds, reflecting the impact of poverty and dietary factors in the aetiology of obesity and diabetes. In the US, the prevalence of childhood diabetes is higher, with a recent estimated population prevalence of 0.67 cases per 1000 children aged between 10 and 19 years.

The high rates of T2DM appearing in children is of particular concern, as evidence is emerging that the natural history of the disease is worse than in later onset T2DM, with very high rates of early microvascular complications. A large study, Treatment Options for Type 2 Diabetes in Adolescents and Youth (TODAY), designed to study the efficacy of treatment for T2DM in young people has provided considerable insight into the severity of the condition. In the TODAY study, the cumulative incidence of any microvascular complication was 50% by 9 years and 80% by 15 years of T2DM duration. Retinopathy was present in 50% of TODAY participants by age 25 years, with a cumulative incidence of nephropathy of 35%. This compares with a prevalence of microvascular complications of around 25% after 10 years of T1DM.

As yet, there is relatively little specific data to guide the management of T2DM in children and young people; as in adult practice, metformin may be considered as a first-line treatment, but there is a paucity of evidence in relation to other oral treatments and many children progress to insulin early in the course of their condition. However, there is increased use of GLP-1 receptor agonists and liraglutide has now obtained a specific license for use in the paediatric age group. Given the association with obesity, the use of GLP-1 agonists is likely to assume an increasingly important role in the management of childhood T2DM.

BIBLIOGRAPHY

Mortensen HB, Hougaard P, The Hvidore Study Group on Childhood Diabetes. Comparison of metabolic control in a cross-sectional study of 2873 children and adolescents with IDDM from 18 countries. Diabetes Care. 1997; 20: 714–20

Northam EA, Matthews LK, Anderson PJ, et al. Psychiatric morbidity and health outcome in type 1 diabetes – Perspectives from a prospective longitudinal study. Diabet Med. 2005; 22: 152–7

Perng W, Conway R, Mayer-Davis E, Dabelea D. Youth-onset type 2 diabetes: The epidemiology of an awakening epidemic. Diabetes Care. 2023 Mar 1; 46(3): 490–99. doi: 10.2337/dci22-0046

Williams RM, Dunger DB. Insulin treatment in children and adolescents. Acta Paediatr. 2004; 93: 440–6

6

Diabetes and surgery: Inpatient and perioperative diabetes care

About 15% of all people admitted to hospital will have diabetes as a comorbidity but, despite this, provision for inpatient management of diabetes is often suboptimal, with poor understanding of diabetes management by generalist hospital staff and variable provision of specialist support. Over the past decade, there have been improvements in this area, with increased recognition of the importance of optimising glucose management to improve outcomes and reduce the length of inpatient stay. In England, the quality of diabetes inpatient care has been tracked by an annual National Diabetes Inpatient Audit (NaDIA) conducted since 2010. The most recent report based on data from 2019 showed an increase in the proportion of people with diabetes seen by specialist teams and a reduction in inpatient hypoglycaemia, but drug errors (particularly in relation to insulin administration) were common and, alarmingly, 3.6% of those with type 1 diabetes mellitus (T1DM) developed ketoacidosis during the course of their admission. There have been delays implementing improvements in diabetes technology in inpatient care, and many patients report frustration around the lack of support for insulin pump treatment and continuous glucose monitoring, with many being obliged to revert to traditional capillary glucose monitoring for the duration of their hospital stay.

Diabetes can have a significant impact on the outcomes of surgical procedures. Recent data have shown that people with diabetes continue to have a significantly longer hospital stays and more postoperative complications, with an estimated excess length of stay of up to 45% than expected for non-diabetic patients undergoing the same procedure. Furthermore, diabetes is associated with a higher risk of critical-care admission in the postoperative period and higher mortality rates. In part, this reflects the comorbidities associated with diabetes, particularly cardiovascular disease and nephropathy which may be exacerbated by surgery. The incidence of perioperative acute kidney injury is higher in patients with diabetes than in the general population and, in some cases, this may reflect the presence of early and previously silent diabetic nephropathy.

Surgery can have a marked effect on blood glucose control and, without adequate management, can lead to acute decompensation of metabolic control. The trauma associated with surgery results in an acute stress response, the magnitude of which depends on the severity of the surgery and the underlying condition, in particular, the presence of infection at the time of surgery (for example in a case of abdominal surgery for a perforated viscus). As part of the stress response, there is an increase in serum cortisol and catecholamines, which impact insulin sensitivity and promote hyperglycaemia and ketone production which, if unchecked, can lead to the development of diabetic ketoacidosis in patients with no or low endogenous insulin secretion.

PERIOPERATIVE MANAGEMENT

Factors to consider in the management of diabetic patients are the severity of surgical trauma and its duration, the pre-existing diabetes treatment and the extent of the patient's endogenous insulin reserves. Patients with T1DM and, for practical

DOI: 10.1201/9781003342700-6

purposes, those with type 2 diabetes mellitus (T2DM) treated with insulin, are assumed to have no endogenous insulin and, will therefore require exogenous insulin administration to cover any surgery. Other patients will only require insulin therapy for major surgery procedures and may be able to continue with oral agents alone for more minor procedures.

Historically, patients with insulin-treated diabetes have been admitted to hospital a day or more before surgery for optimisation and preoperative insulin management. While this may be required for some patients with poor glycaemic control or where prolonged fasting is required, most patients can be admitted on the day of surgery, and diabetes is no longer considered to be a contraindication to day case surgical treatment.

The aim of management of diabetes during surgery is to maintain stable glucose levels close to the normal range, avoiding marked glucose excursions and, in particular, avoiding hypoglycaemia. There is consensus that an appropriate target glucose range is 6–10 mmol/l (108–180 mg/dl), with acceptance of upwards excursion to 12 mmol/l (216 mg/dl). Glucose levels much above this should be avoided, as they may impact wound healing, and there is some evidence of an association between perioperative hyperglycaemia and postoperative infection rates.

PATIENTS ON NON-INSULIN TREATMENT

When pre-existing glycaemic control is acceptable on oral agents or glucagon-like peptide-1 (GLP-1) agonist treatment and minor surgery is planned, patients can usually be managed safely by fasting and the omission of the usual oral medication on the day of the procedure. For some drugs, cessation in the days before surgery is desirable. Longer-acting sulphonylureas are best omitted on the day prior to surgery to reduce the risk of any residual action and associated hypoglycaemia. SGLT-2 inhibitors should also be discontinued to reduce the risk of ketosis associated with the use of this class of agents in the presence of a stress response, and it is generally recommended that these are stopped 3 to 4 days before surgery. For procedures that involve the use of contrast dye, it is also recommended that metformin is discontinued 24 to 48 hours before surgery.

SGLT-2 and metformin should only be restarted when normal oral fluid and dietary intake is established. For non-insulin-treated patients, glucose infusions should be avoided and blood glucose checked hourly during surgery and the early perioperative phase. In the event of a sustained glucose rise above the upper target limit of 12 mmol/l, insulin and glucose substrate solution should be started, as detailed later in the chapter, for patients on insulin treatment. Postoperatively, oral agents may be recommenced at the time of the next meal. When glycaemic control is poor or major surgery is planned, it is desirable to admit the patient before the day of operation to optimise blood glucose control with short- or intermediate-acting insulins. On the day of surgery, breakfast is omitted and the surgery covered with intravenous (IV) insulin and glucose (discussed later). Postoperatively, subcutaneous insulin is continued until blood glucose levels are stable when the patient can restart oral therapy.

PATIENTS ON INSULIN THERAPY

The principle behind insulin management during surgery is to maintain near normoglycaemia with avoidance of hypoglycaemia and to maintain normal electrolyte balance. To achieve this, current guidance recommends the use of a variable-rate insulin infusion delivered by a syringe driver infused alongside a balanced substrate solution containing both sodium and glucose. This is in contrast to older regimes which advocated adding insulin and potassium to infusion bags of 5% or 10% glucose, as these regimes do not allow adequate adjustment of insulin to maintain optimal glucose control, and the use of glucose as the sole substrate risks causing hyponatraemia. The current recommended substrate solution for surgical management is 0.45% saline with 5% glucose and 0.15% to 0.3% potassium chloride (depending on baseline potassium levels). As an alternative, 4% glucose in 0.18% saline and 0.15%/0.3% potassium chloride is recommended when the former is not available. For those patients on long-acting basal insulin analogues (e.g. insulin glargine, detemir or degludec), it is recommended that the basal insulin is continued pre- and postoperatively, but at a reduced dose calculated as 80% of the usual basal insulin requirement. Continuing the basal insulin facilitates switching back to subcutaneous insulin when normal feeding resumes and reduces the need for higher-dose IV insulin treatment in the perioperative period.

It is recommended that the regime is started at the time of induction of surgery or at the time of the first missed meal if there is any prolongation of preoperative fasting. IV insulin and glucose substrate should normally be continued until oral intake is resumed.

PATIENTS ON INSULIN PUMP TREATMENT

Patients established on insulin pump treatment can usually be managed effectively by continuing to use this during surgery and the perioperative period to reduce the need for IV insulin, particularly for more minor procedures. In preparation for surgery, it is desirable to ensure optimisation of basal pump rates by assessing the response to performing a limited fast a day prior to surgery and determining that glucose remains stable on basal insulin in the absence of mealtime boluses. If there is any tendency to a downward drift in glucose, consideration should be given to reducing the basal rate to around 80% of usual treatment dose. Continuing with subcutaneous insulin-pump treatment has the advantage of allowing a more rapid return to usual treatment than switching to an IV regime. However, there is less opportunity to make adjustments to treatment than with IV insulin treatment and, thus, for more major procedures, switching to

an IV insulin and substrate regime may be more appropriate.

BIBLIOGRAPHY

Dhatariya K, Levy N. Perioperative diabetes care. Clin Med (Lond). 2019 Nov; 19(6): 437–40. doi: 10.7861/clinmed.2019.0226

Diabetes Guideline Working Group, Centre for Perioperative Care. Guideline for Perioperatieve Care for people with Diabetes Mellitus Undergoing Elective and Emergency Surgery. Published online March 2021 at: https://www.cpoc.org.uk/sites/cpoc/files/documents/2021-03/CPOC-Guideline for Perioperative Care for People with Diabetes Mellitus Undergoing Elective and Emergency Surgery.pdf

NHS Digital. National Diabetes Inpatient Audit Report 2019. Published online at https://files.digital.nhs.uk/F6/49FA05/NaDIA%202019%20-%20Full%20Report%20v1.1.pdf

Partridge H, Perkins B, Mathieu S, et al. Clinical recommendations in the management of the patient with type 1 diabetes on insulin pump therapy in the perioperative period. Br J Anaesth. 2016: 116, 18–26. https://doi.org/10.1093/bja/aev347

Sudhakaran S, Surani SR. Guidelines for perioperative management of the diabetic patient. Surg Res Pract. 2015; 2015: 284063. doi: 10.1155/2015/284063

7

Acute complications of diabetes

HYPOGLYCAEMIA

Hypoglycaemia is the greatest fear of diabetic patients treated with insulin. Hypoglycaemia in patients with type 1 diabetes mellitus (T1DM) is a major source of disruption to their lives

(Figures 7.1 and 7.2). Hypoglycaemia also occurs in patients with type 2 diabetes mellitus (T2DM) treated with sulphonylureas or insulin, although to a lesser extent. The definition of hypoglycaemia is a reduction in the plasma glucose concentration to a level that may induce symptoms or signs such

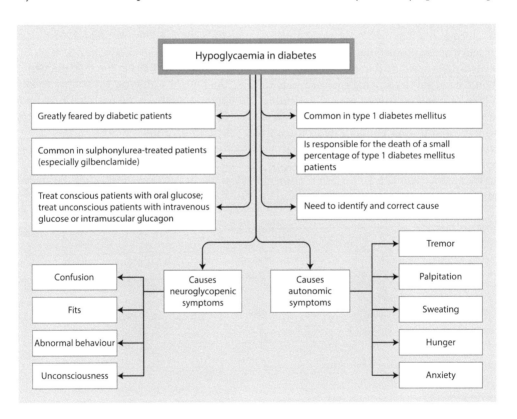

Figure 7.1 Hypoglycaemia is a major problem for insulin-treated diabetic patients; more than 30% of such patients experience hypoglycaemic coma at least once. About 10% experience coma in any given year and around 3% are incapacitated by frequent severe episodes. Hypoglycaemia is usually due to an excessive dose of insulin, reduced or delayed ingestion of food, or increased energy expenditure owing to exercise. Identification of the cause and appropriate remedial action and education are mandatory. Patients treated with sulphonylureas frequently experience hypoglycaemia.

DOI: 10.1201/9781003342700-7

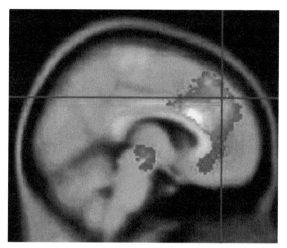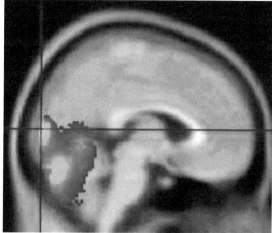

Figure 7.2 Hypoglycaemia is associated with regional brain activation. Here, CMG positron emission tomography (PET) has been used to measure changes in global and regional brain glucose metabolism. Hypoglycaemia has been shown to be associated with activation of the brain stem, prefrontal cortex and anterior cingulate (yellow/orange indicates regions of increased glucose uptake and metabolism) and with reduced neuronal activation in the midline occipital cortex and cerebellar vermis (blue).

as altered mental status and/or sympathetic system stimulation. Numerically, there is no universal agreement as to the actual glucose concentration below which hypoglycaemia exists (especially as the glucose concentration below which symptoms emerge varies from individual to individual), but, generally, hypoglycaemia is defined as a glucose level below 3.9 mmol/L (70 mg/dl). Acute hypoglycaemia produces autonomic symptoms (such as sweating, tremor, palpitations and hunger) or neuroglycopaenic symptoms (impaired cognitive function, such as difficulty in concentrating and incoordination). If neuroglycopaenic symptoms occur without prior warning of autonomic symptoms (hypoglycaemic unawareness), unconsciousness and/or seizures may develop. Death from hypoglycaemia is rare (estimated at 2–4% of patients with T1DM) and is often associated with the excessive use of alcohol or with deliberate insulin overdose. Unexpected deaths, thought to be attributable to hypoglycaemia, are reported in young people with T1DM who are usually found dead in bed. Such deaths may be caused by hypoglycaemia-induced cardiac dysrhythmia, although this remains unproven. The average individual patient with T1DM will experience one to two episodes of symptomatic hypoglycaemia per week and may experience one or more temporarily disabling hypoglycaemic events requiring third-party assistance per year. Hypoglycaemia also occurs in

patients with T2DM, especially those treated with insulin. In a meta-analysis of studies incorporating 532,542 people with T2DM on oral therapies and insulin, the prevalence of mild/moderate hypoglycaemia was 45% and severe hypoglycaemia was 6%. The incidence of hypoglycaemic episodes per person-year for mild/moderate and for severe was 19 and 0.80, respectively. The prevalence and incidence rates were higher for insulin-treated patients, while patients on sulphonylureas had higher rates than those not treated with a sulphonylurea. The main causes of hypoglycaemia are excessive doses of insulin or sulphonylureas, inadequate or delayed ingestion of food and sudden or prolonged exercise.

Hypoglycaemia is usually self-treated by the ingestion of glucose tablets (15–20 g) or carbohydrate or a meal. The 15-15 Rule is a useful guide (Figure 7.3). The patient should consume 15 g of glucose or carbohydrate then wait 15 minutes before testing their blood glucose again. If the glucose level is still <3.9 mmol/L (70 mg/dl), the exercise should be repeated until the blood glucose rises to above 3.9 mmol/L (70 mg/dl). At that point, a snack or meal should be ingested. Some guidelines include the use of 40% glucose gel (Glucogel, Dextrogel, Rapilose) smeared into the mouth. If the patient is unable to ingest glucose, then glucagon 1.0 mg in a powder for reconstitution (Glucagon Emergency Kit, Eli Lilly; GlucaGen HypoKit,

---

AMERICAN DIABETES ASSOCIATION TREATMENT OF HYPOGLYCAEMIA: THE '15-15 RULE'

Have 15 grams of carbohydrate to raise your blood glucose.

Check blood glucose after 15 minutes.

If it is still below 70 mg/dl (3.9 mmol/l), take another 15 gram serving.

Repeat these steps until your blood glucose is at least 70 mg/dl (3.9 mmol/l).

Once your glucose is back to normal, eat a meal or snack to make sure it doesn't fall again.

Figure 7.3 The 15-15 Rule for the treatment of hypoglycaemia.

Novo Nordisk) should be injected subcutaneously or intramuscularly. Glucagon enhances hepatic glucose production by promoting glycogenolysis and gluconeogenesis while inhibiting glycolysis. Newer formulations of glucagon are now available in some countries and include a nasal preparation of glucagon, Baqsimi Nasal Powder (Eli Lilly), and pre-filled syringes and autoinjectors containing a liquid formulation of glucagon: Gvoke and Gvoke HypoPen (US, Xeris Pharmaceuticals Inc) (Figure 7.4), Ogluo (UK/EU, Tetris Pharma Ltd) and Zegalogue (dasiglucagon, Zealand Pharma). These are useful adjuncts to the treatment of hypoglycaemia for diabetic patients. Unconscious patients in hospital can be treated intravenously with 75–100 ml of 20% glucose or 150–200 ml 10% glucose over 15 minutes followed by a 10% infusion.

Patients experiencing recurrent hypoglycaemia need to liaise with their medical or specialist nursing advisors to determine the cause and to establish appropriate measures of prevention. When patients experience hypoglycaemic unawareness, a strategy of loosening blood-glucose control with strict avoidance of low blood-glucose levels (<3.9 mmol/L, 70 mg/dl) is advised and has been shown to be associated with a resumption of awareness of hypoglycaemia.

Recurrent hypoglycaemia and hypoglycaemic unawareness pose particular problems for drivers and for those engaged in certain high-risk occupations, e.g. operating heavy machinery. Patients should be advised to avoid such activities until these problems can be eliminated with the help of the diabetic team.

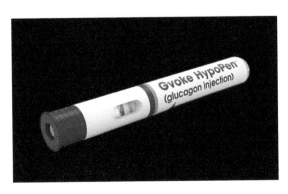 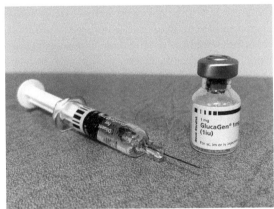

Figure 7.4 GvokeHypoPen, a pre-filled autoinjector containing a liquid formulation for the treatment of hypoglycaemia (left). Glucagon as GlucaGen 1 mg (1 iu) for subcutaneous, intramuscular or intravenous injection (right).

DIABETIC KETOACIDOSIS AND HYPEROSMOLAR HYPERGLYCAEMIC STATE

Biochemically, diabetic ketoacidosis (DKA) is present when blood ketones are >5 mEq/L (or urinary ketones are greater than or equal to 3+), plasma glucose is >13.9 mmol/L (250 mg/dl), although it can be less in particular circumstances, and the blood arterial pH is <7.3, associated with a low serum bicarbonate of 18 mmol/L (18 mEq/L) or less and an increase in the anion gap. Thus, DKA is characterized by hyperglycaemia, hyperketonaemia with ketonuria and metabolic acidosis (Figure 7.5). DKA occurs as a consequence of absolute or relative insulin deficiency accompanied by an increase in counter-regulatory hormones (cortisol, glucagon, growth hormone, epinephrine) resulting in increased hepatic gluconeogenesis, glycolysis and lipolysis. Severe hyperglycaemia ensues while the breakdown of fat generates increasing levels of ketones and ketoacids which overwhelm the body's ability to buffer them, leading to acidosis. Glycosuria leads to osmotic diuresis, dehydration and hyperosmolarity. Potassium loss is caused by a shift of potassium from the extracellular space to the intracellular space in exchange with extracellular hydrogen ions.

DKA accounts for the majority of deaths in young people with T1DM (while cardiovascular disease and end-stage renal failure are largely responsible for deaths in people with longstanding T1DM). The most common cause of DKA is infection followed by missed or disrupted insulin administration and new, previously undiagnosed, T1DM (Figure 7.6). Most cases of DKA occur in young people. DKA may occasionally be seen in patients with T2DM (especially in patients with 'ketosis-prone' T2DM), and the usual precipitant is myocardial infarction or other major concomitant illness. DKA in pregnancy is an even greater medical emergency as both mother and fetus are at risk. Recurrent DKA is frequently seen in young women with T1DM where the causative factor is usually insulin omission. In some instances, no clear discernible cause is found.

DKA is characterised clinically by symptoms of nausea, vomiting, thirst, polyuria and, occasionally, abdominal pain accompanied by signs of dehydration, acidotic respiration, ketones on the breath, hypothermia and altered consciousness.

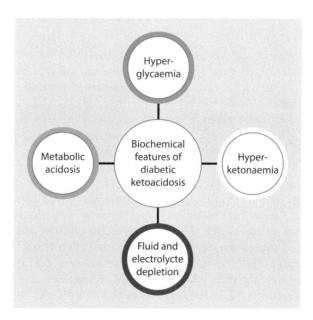

Figure 7.5 Diabetic ketoacidosis remains a significant cause of death in patients with type 1 diabetes mellitus and is characterized by marked hyperglycaemia, hyperketonaemia (usually detected by the presence of ketonuria), a low arterial pH and fluid and electrolyte depletion with prerenal uraemia. Treatment involves rehydration with saline, low-dose intravenous insulin infusion, potassium replacement, and therapy directed at the underlying cause, if apparent.

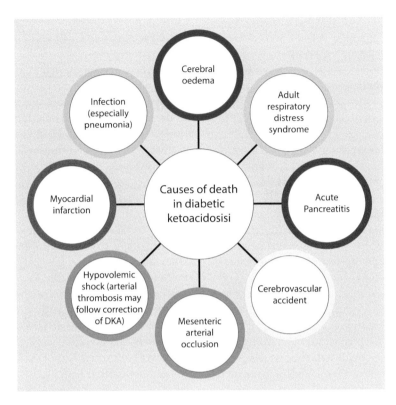

Figure 7.6 Myocardial infarction and infection are the most common causes of death in diabetic ketoacidosis. Cerebral oedema is an uncommon and poorly understood cause of death, and appears to have a predilection for younger patients. Thromboembolic complications are an important cause of mortality.

Detailed biochemical assessment and monitoring (of renal function, electrolytes, glucose and arterial gases) are mandatory in the management of this condition, and a search should be undertaken for the underlying cause (by chest radiography, urine and blood cultures, etc.). If a treatable underlying cause is found, it should be treated promptly.

Successful treatment of DKA necessitates vigorous fluid replacement, correction of potassium deficiency, continuous intravenous insulin infusion, attention to acid–base status and treatment of the underlying cause where identifiable. Fluid replacement is the vital first step in management, followed by insulin treatment. Fluid replacement should be with 0.9% sodium chloride solution (typical fluid replacement regimen 1 L in the first hour, 2 L next 4 hours, 2 L in next 8 hours for a 70 kg adult). If the initial systolic blood pressure is <90 mm Hg, then 500 ml of 0.9% sodium chloride solution should be administered over 10–15 minutes (this may need to be repeated). No potassium should be given if the initial plasma potassium is >5.5 mmol/L (5.5 mEq/L). Thereafter, 40 mmol (40 mEq) of potassium should be added to each litre of the sodium chloride solution, usually in a premixed bag, and adjusted accordingly. Insulin is administered via a fixed-rate intravenous insulin infusion at a rate of 0.1 units/kg body weight/hour (the patient's body weight may need to be estimated). When the plasma glucose level falls below 14 mmol/L (252 mg/dl), an infusion of 10% dextrose should be commenced, usually to run concurrently with the sodium chloride solution. The insulin infusion rate may need to be halved to 0.05 units/kg/h to avoid the risk of hypoglycaemia. If the patient was on a long-acting insulin, then this should be continued. Pump-treated patients should have their continuous subcutaneous insulin infusion stopped temporarily. The administration of bicarbonate (or phosphate) is not recommended routinely. The aim of treatment is to reduce blood ketones by 0.5 mmol/L/h (5.0 mg/dl/h), the venous bicarbonate by 3.0 mmol/L/h (3.0 mEq/L/h), the plasma glucose by 3.0 mmol/L/h (54 mg/dl/h) and to maintain the potassium between 4.0 and 5.5 mmol/L (4.0–5.5 mEq/L). To achieve this necessitates frequent biochemical monitoring of glucose, capillary ketones, venous pH or bicarbonate and potassium. Once the patient is stabilised, the involvement of the specialist diabetic team should be sought to commence or adjust the patient's usual insulin regime and to seek to determine what factors led to DKA in the first place and how they could be prevented in future. The in-patient mortality from DKA in the US and the UK is less than 1%. The overall mortality is approximately 0.2–2.0%, but is 5% in those under 40 years of age and may be approaching 20% in the elderly or those with serious concomitant illness. Cerebral oedema, especially in children, is a rare (0.2–1% of cases), serious and unexplained complication of DKA and may respond to intravenous mannitol or dexamethasone. Children with DKA should be treated according to paediatric DKA treatment protocols.

An important variant of DKA is euglycaemic diabetic ketoacidosis (EDKA), characterised by euglycaemia (glucose <13.9 mmol/L, 250 mg/dl), severe metabolic acidosis (pH <7.3, bicarbonate <18 mmol/L (18 mEq/L) and ketonaemia. The overall mechanism is based on a general state of starvation, resulting in ketosis while maintaining normoglycaemia. Thus, it is associated with anorexia, gastroparesis, fasting and alcohol misuse. Trigger factors may be pregnancy, pancreatitis, surgery, infection, cocaine toxicity, cirrhosis and insulin-pump use. The use of SGLT2 (sodium-glucose cotransporter-2) inhibitors such as canagliflozin, dapagliflozin and empagliflozin can also result in EDKA. Treatment is directed at fluid resuscitation, insulin infusion and the co-administration of 5–10% dextrose. The normal blood-glucose levels at presentation may delay the diagnosis of this serious acidotic condition.

Hyperosmolar Hyperglycaemic State (HHS)

Hyperosmolar Hyperglycaemic State (HHS) is also known as Hyperosmolar Hyperglycaemic Nonketotic Syndrome (HHNS) and was previously known as Hyperglycaemic Hyperosmolar Nonketotic Coma (HONK). HHS is one further life-threatening metabolic derangement which occurs in diabetes most commonly in patients with T2DM (Figure 7.7). The mortality rate for HHS far exceeds that of DKA, reaching up to 5–10%. Coma is found in fewer than 20% of patients with HHS, hence, the abandonment of the term HONK. HHS is characterised by hyperosmolarity, severe hyperglycaemia and dehydration without significant ketoacidosis and is most commonly encountered in patients with T2DM with concomitant illness. Patients may present with focal or global neurological deficits. The basic underlying problem with HHS is a relative reduction in effective circulating insulin with a concomitant increase in counter-regulatory hormones. Ketoacidosis does not develop in HHS, as insulin levels remain adequate to inhibit lipolysis, thereby preventing the generation of ketones. Hyperglycaemia-driven osmotic diuresis results in dehydration with loss of electrolytes such as sodium and potassium. Associated hyperosmolarity and hypotension may ultimately lead to renal shutdown, the end stage of which can be coma and death. The potential causative factors in the development of HHS are multiple, but the majority of cases are due to infection. Any significant illness such as myocardial infarction or pulmonary embolism may trigger HHS, as may concomitant drug therapy, alcohol, withdrawal of oral hypoglycaemic agents or insulin and neglect. Several different ethnic groups, such as African Americans, Hispanics and Native Americans, are disproportionately affected by HHS, but this may just reflect the prevalence of T2DM in these groups. Patients presenting with HHS require extensive investigations to assess their metabolic state as well as tests to look for the precipitating illness, which may include brain imaging if there is an altered conscious level, to exclude intracranial pathology. As the fluid deficit in patients with HHS is of the order of 9 L, aggressive fluid resuscitation with 0.9% sodium chloride solution is the cornerstone of the initial treatment of HHS at a rate of 15–20 mL/kg/h, together with potassium replacement as for DKA. Treatment with 0.45% sodium chloride solution should only be used if the serum osmolarity fails to decline. Once fluid therapy has been initiated, an intravenous insulin infusion can be commenced at a rate of 0.5–0.1 units/kg/h. Insulin should not be administered initially as it may cause a sudden precipitous fall in osmolarity, leading to cardiovascular collapse. Further alterations in the administration of fluids, insulin and potassium should be made on the basis of subsequent frequent monitoring and assessment, preferably undertaken in an ICU.

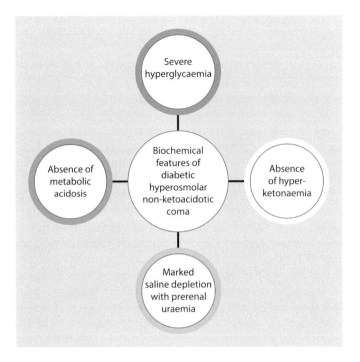

Figure 7.7 Hyperosmolar Hyperglycaemic Syndrome usually affects middle-aged or elderly patients with previously undiagnosed type 2 diabetes mellitus. It is characterized by marked hyperglycaemia (usually >50 mmol/l; 900 mg/dl) and prerenal uraemia without significant hyperketonaemia and acidosis. Treatment is by fluid replacement, attention to electrolyte balance and insulin therapy as for diabetic ketoacidosis, and most patients will not ultimately require permanent insulin therapy. The condition has a high mortality, owing to a high incidence of serious associated disorders and complications.

As there is an increased risk of venous thromboembolism in HHS, all patients should receive treatment with low molecular weight heparin unless there is a contraindication.

BIBLIOGRAPHY

Cryer PE. The barrier of hypoglycemia in diabetes. Diabetes. 2008 Dec; 57(12): 3169–76. Doi: 10.2337/db08-1084

Cryer PE, Fisher JN, Shamoon H. Hypoglycemia. Diabetes Care. 1994; 17: 734–55

Edridge CL, Dunkley AJ, Bodicoat DH, Rose TC, Gray LJ, Davies MJ, Khunti K. Prevalence and incidence of hypoglycaemia in 532,542 people with type 2 diabetes on oral therapies and insulin: A systematic review and meta-analysis of population based studies. PloS One. Doi: 10.1371/journal.pone.0126427

Evans K. Diabetic ketoacidosis: Update on management. Clin Med. 2019 Sep; 19(5): 396–8. Doi: 10.7861/clinmed.2019-0284

Frier BM, Fisher BM, eds. Hypoglycemia and Diabetes. London: Edward Arnold, 1993

Kitabchi AE, Umpierrez GE, Murphy MB, et al. Management of hyperglycaemic crises in patients with diabetes. Diabetes Care. 2001; 24: 131–53

Munro JF, Campbell IW, MacCuish AC, Duncan LJ. Euglycaemic diabetic ketoacidosis. Br Med J. 1973 Jun 9; 2(5866): 578–80. Doi: 10.1136/bmj.2.5866.578

Schade DS, Eaton RP, Alberti KGGM, Johnston DG. Diabetic Coma: Ketoacidotic and Hyperosmolar. Albuquerque: University of New Mexico Press, 1981

Small M, Alzaid A, MacCuish AC. Diabetic hyperosmolar non-ketoacidotic decompensation. Q J Med. 1988; 66: 251–7

Umpierrez GE, Murphy MB, Kitabchi AE. Diabetic ketoacidosis and hyperglycemic hyperosmolar syndrome. Diabetes Spectr. 2002; 15(1): 28–36. Doi: 10.2337/diaspect.15.1.28

8

Chronic complications of diabetes

Although the acute complications of diabetes impact significantly the day-to-day life of people with diabetes, especially type 1 diabetes mellitus (T1DM), the knowledge of the potential risk of chronic complications is ever present. Results from the Diabetes Control and Complications Trial (DCCT) established unequivocally the relationship between glycaemic control and the incidence and progression of diabetic microvascular complications. Such complications occur in both T1DM and type 2 diabetes mellitus (T2DM) patients, although the latter patients often succumb to major cardiovascular disease before microvascular complications become advanced. Although life expectancy for T1DM patients is undoubtedly reduced, more than 40% of such patients will survive for more than 40 years, half of them without developing significant microvascular complications. The United Kingdom Prospective Diabetes Study (UKPDS) also provided pivotal information on the relationship between glucose control and complications in T2DM patients. It demonstrated, in a significant way, the beneficial effect of an improvement in blood glucose control on subsequent risk of developing specific diabetic complications.

DIABETIC RETINOPATHY

Both the incidence and prevalence of diabetic retinopathy are highest in T1DM patients with an early age of onset of diabetes. However, T1DM patients do not exhibit retinopathy at presentation, and the likelihood of developing significant diabetic eye disease in the first 5 years of the disease is small. In contrast, T2DM patients may have retinopathy at presentation, presumably because they have had previously unrecognised T2DM for many years. The prevalence of retinopathy increases with the duration of diabetes. In general, significant visual impairment is usually caused by proliferative retinopathy in T1DM and by maculopathy in T2DM. Diabetic retinopathy is the leading cause of new blindness in persons aged 25–74 years in the US. The estimated prevalence of diabetic retinopathy is 28.5% among those with diabetes aged 40 years and over.

Background diabetic retinopathy (Figures 8.1–8.8) is characterised by capillary dilatation and occlusion, microaneurysms, 'dot and blot' haemorrhages, flame-shaped haemorrhages, retinal

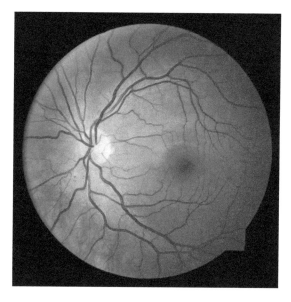

Figure 8.1 Normal fundus of the eye. Appreciation of the fundal abnormalities seen in diabetes must be based on a sound knowledge of the normal appearance.

DOI: 10.1201/9781003342700-8

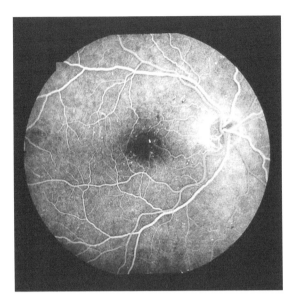

Figure 8.2 Optic atrophy in diabetes insipidus, diabetes mellitus, optic atrophy and deafness (DIDMOAD) syndrome, a rare condition that is usually diagnosed when type 1 diabetes mellitus (T1DM) presents in childhood. The inheritance is autosomal recessive and diabetes insipidus tends to develop after the diagnosis of T1DM.

Figure 8.4 The fluorescein angiogram of the same area as in Figure 8.3 reveals many more abnormalities than can be seen on the fundal photograph. Widespread microaneurysms appear as white dots.

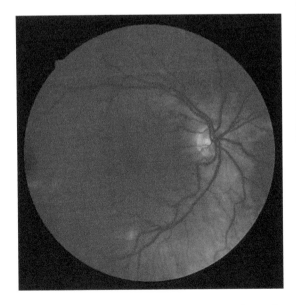

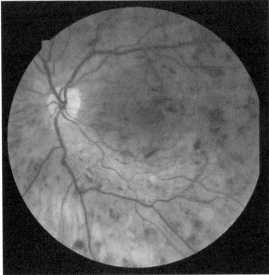

Figure 8.5 Severe background diabetic retinopathy includes venous changes, clusters and large blot haemorrhages, intraretinal microvascular abnormalities (IRMA), an early cottonwool spot and a generally ischaemic appearance. This type of retinopathy is usually a prelude to proliferative change.

Figure 8.3 Background diabetic retinopathy with occasional scattered microaneurysms and dot haemorrhages.

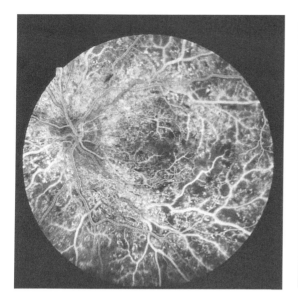

Figure 8.6 A fluorescein angiogram of the same area as in Figure 8.5 shows the blind ends of occluded small vessels, widespread capillary leakage and areas of non-perfusion.

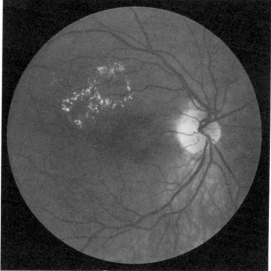

Figure 8.8 Circinate exudative retinopathy. The two hard exudate rings (lateral to the macula) are true exudates due to leakage from abnormal vessels and are associated with retinal oedema. When hard exudates and retinal oedema affect the macular area, the fovea may become involved, which may threaten central vision. Laser photocoagulation helps to prevent such loss of vision.

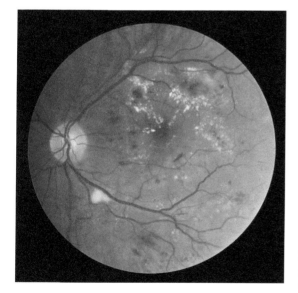

Figure 8.7 Serious diabetic retinopathy with venous irregularities, blot haemorrhages, intraretinal microvascular abnormalities, large cottonwool spots and extensive areas of hard exudates.

oedema and hard exudates (which are true exudates of lipid-rich material from abnormal vessels). This picture represents non-proliferative retinopathy and is not associated with visual loss unless hard exudates become extensive and involve the fovea. Preproliferative lesions, a harbinger of impending new vessel formation, include cottonwool spots (nerve-fibre layer infarctions caused by occlusion of precapillary arterioles), venous loops and beading, arterial narrowing and occlusion and intraretinal microvascular abnormalities. The latter consist of abnormal dilated capillaries, which are often leaky.

The importance of the recognition of preproliferative retinopathy is that it indicates the need for urgent referral to an ophthalmologist. In proliferative retinopathy (Figures 8.9–8.12) new vessels originate from a major vein (occasionally from arteries) and appear in the retinal periphery or on the optic disc. They are much less common in T2DM than in T1DM. New vessels have a devastating impact on vision when they burst and produce sudden preretinal or vitreous haemorrhage. Contraction of associated fibroglial tissue may result in retinal detachment with resultant

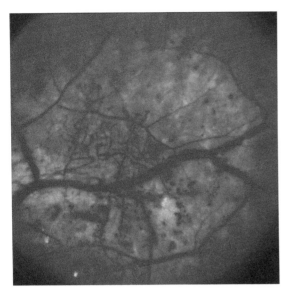

Figure 8.9 Serious gross peripheral proliferative diabetic retinopathy includes marked venous changes such as dilatation and beading.

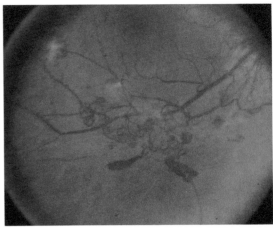

Figure 8.11 Leashes of peripheral new vessels with associated haemorrhage. These lesions are amenable to laser photocoagulation.

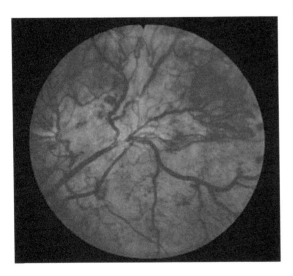

Figure 8.10 Extensive peripheral proliferative retinopathy with venous beading and blot haemorrhages. New vessels usually originate from a major vein and adopt a branching pattern. Proliferative retinopathy is the most common sight-threatening complication of type 1 diabetes mellitus, with visual loss being due to breakage of vessels leading to preretinal or vitreous haemorrhage. It is always accompanied by other diabetic lesions and is treatable by laser photocoagulation. It is less common in type 2 diabetes mellitus (where exudative maculopathy is the most common cause of visual loss).

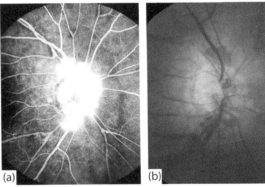

Figure 8.12 Fluorescein angiogram (A) and fundal photograph (B) of new vessels at the optic disc, which lead rapidly to visual loss. If haemorrhage has already occurred, then visual loss is imminent and urgent laser treatment is indicated. Fluorescein angiography reveals the gross leakage from the abnormal vessels.

loss of vision, which may be profound if it affects the macula (Figures 8.13, 8.14).

Diabetic maculopathy is the most common cause of visual loss in T2DM and may be exudative, oedematous or ischaemic. If left untreated, preproliferative retinopathy, proliferative retinopathy and maculopathy will all have an appalling prognosis for the patient's eyesight. All diabetic patients should be regularly screened for such changes and referred, where appropriate, for specialised ophthalmic assessment.

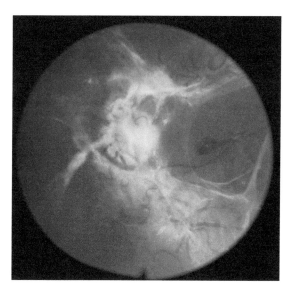

Figure 8.13 End-stage diabetic retinopathy is characterised by gross distortion of the retina with extensive fibrous bands. Uncontrolled new vessels develop a fibrous tissue covering and expanding fibrous tissue tends to contract, causing retinal traction and detachment. The result is sudden and unexpected visual loss. The retinopathy shown here is untreatable.

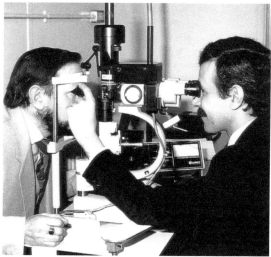

Figure 8.15 A patient undergoing laser photocoagulation for diabetic retinopathy. A high-energy light beam is focused through a corneal contact lens onto the target area of the retina. Laser photocoagulation can be used to destroy specific targets (e.g. peripheral new vessels) or to perform panretinal photocoagulation.

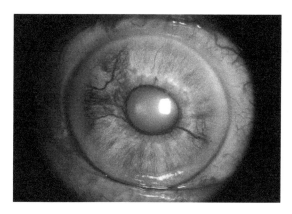

Figure 8.14 In profoundly ischaemic diabetic eyes, thromboneovascular glaucoma may occur with new vessel and fibrous tissue proliferation in the angle of the anterior chamber, which interferes with normal aqueous drainage. The condition is associated with rubeosis iridis (shown here) wherein new vessel growth occurs on the iris.

Laser photocoagulation (Figures 8.15) can be used to destroy isolated new vessels or to undertake panretinal photocoagulation in cases of more severe proliferative retinopathy. The aim of the panretinal approach is to reduce retinal ischaemia overall, thereby reducing the stimulus to new vessel formation (Figure 8.16). Photocoagulation may also be used for the treatment of diabetic macular oedema, with focal treatment given for discrete lesions and diffuse treatment for widespread capillary leakage and non-perfusion. Intravitreal injection of vascular endothelial growth factor (VEGF) inhibitors such as bevacizumab, ranibizumab, brolucizumab, faricimab and aflibercept is now the preferred treatment for central-involved macular oedema, with most patients requiring near-monthly intravitreal therapy in the first year. VEGF inhibitor therapy is also an effective treatment of proliferative diabetic retinopathy. Intravitreal triamcinolone (or an intravitreal dexamethasone implant—Ozurdex) may be employed in the treatment of diabetic macular oedema, proliferative diabetic retinopathy and neovascular glaucoma as a consequence of proliferative retinopathy and has been found to be effective in reducing central macular thickness and improving visual acuity (Figures 8.17–8.19). It may also have an antiangiogenic effect. In advanced cases, vitreoretinal surgery, including vitrectomy, may need to be performed to treat

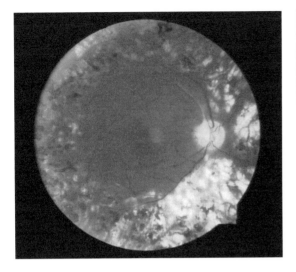

Figure 8.16 Panretinal laser photocoagulation. The entire retina is treated except for the macula and papillomacular bundle, which are essential for central vision. The rationale for using photocoagulation in proliferative retinopathy is that it destroys the ischaemic areas of the retina which produce vasoproliferative factors that stimulate new vessel growth. Panretinal photocoagulation may require 1500–2000 burns. The treatment is well tolerated and divided into several sessions, and regression of new vessels is usually seen within 3–4 weeks. Once the treatment is effective, the results are long-lasting. In maculopathy, laser treatment is either focused on discrete lesions or uses a diffuse 'grid' treatment in cases of widespread capillary leakage and non-perfusion. However, treatment is less effective and the long-term outlook is not as good.

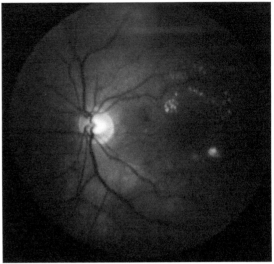

Figure 8.18 The same retina as in Figure 8.17 at 3 months postintravitreal triamcinolone therapy. The changes are not dramatic, but there is an improvement with partial resolution of hard exudates around the macula. The role of intravitreal triamcinolone therapy has not been fully established; however, some retina specialists use it to treat diabetic macular oedema which persists despite laser therapy. It is not a substitute for laser therapy and one recent study showed it had only a marginal benefit over the long term, while increasing the incidence of cataract and glaucoma.

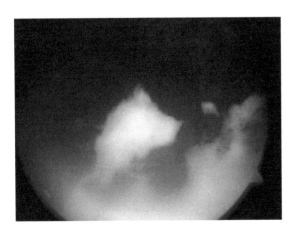

Figure 8.17 Triamcinolone has been inserted into the vitreous under topical anaesthesia in a patient with diabetic maculopathy.

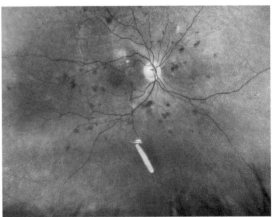

Figure 8.19 This is the retinal photograph of a 77-year-old pseudophakic diabetic female with severe bilateral diabetic macular oedema refractory to anti-vascular endothelial growth factor (anti-VEGF) with an Ozurdex implant in situ, resulting in improved visual acuity.

severe vitreous haemorrhage and retinal detachment (Figures 8.20–8.22).

Detection of diabetic retinopathy at an early stage is essential. All diabetic patients should have a regular ophthalmic examination, with patients

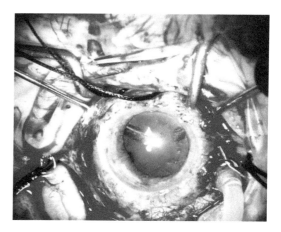

Figure 8.22 Severe vitreous haemorrhage may lead to secondary retinal detachment. Although vitrectomy may be performed electively for severe vitreous haemorrhage alone, urgent surgery is required for operable retinal detachment. Vitreoretinal microsurgery requires a closed intraocular approach (shown here). An operating microscope allows precise intraocular manipulation to remove the vitreous and its contained haemorrhage, which is replaced with saline and followed by endolaser photocoagulation to prevent both further detachment and subsequent neovascularisation.

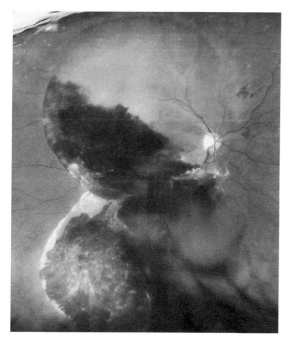

Figure 8.20 Vitreous haemorrhage has occurred despite extensive laser photocoagulation. The haemorrhage may clear but, if it fails to do so or recurrent haemorrhage ensues, visual loss is inevitable and vitreoretinal surgery may be indicated.

with T1DM having a comprehensive eye examination within 5 years of diagnosis and patients with T2DM having an examination at the time of diagnosis. Screening programmes for retinopathy should be designed to include all patients with diabetes in an attempt to avoid visual loss. The combination of direct ophthalmoscopy and digital retinal photography with measurement of visual acuity is often used. Suitably qualified optometrists have also been employed in some screening programmes (Figure 8.23).

DIABETIC NEPHROPATHY

Diabetic nephropathy, one of the most serious complications of diabetes, is characterised by proteinuria, decreasing glomerular filtration rate and increasing blood pressure. In the absence of urinary infection or other renal disease, diabetic nephropathy is defined by the detection of albuminuria of 300 mg/day or greater (200 micrograms/minute) or an albumin-to-creatinine ratio (ACR) greater than 300 mg/g (30 mg/mmol) on two occasions 3–6 months apart. In patients with T1DM, when

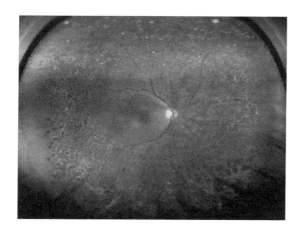

Figure 8.21 The same patient as in Figure 8.20 postvitrectomy with resultant clearing of the vitreous haemorrhage.

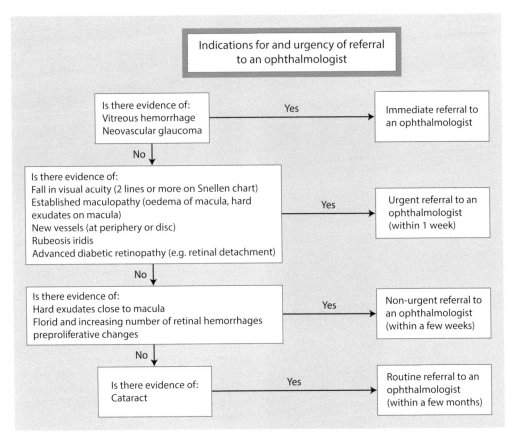

Figure 8.23 Once diabetic retinopathy has been identified, referral to an ophthalmologist may be indicated. This chart shows the types of diabetic eye disease requiring such referral and the urgency with which it should be undertaken.

this degree of proteinuria is associated with the presence of established diabetic retinopathy, the histology of the underlying kidneys will inevitably be that of diabetic glomerulopathy, although, in T2DM, nephropathy can exist without concomitant retinopathy. This degree of proteinuria is detectable by dipstick urine testing. However, it is recognised that this stage is preceded by a long phase of incipient nephropathy associated with microalbuminuria (30–300 mg/day; 30–299 mg/g creatinine) that is not detectable on dipstick testing. As microalbuminuria presages diabetic nephropathy, most national guidelines recommend screening for the presence of microalbuminuria annually by measurement of the ACR, allowing the institution of interventional treatment to slow the rate of progression of nephropathy. Histologically, the diabetic kidney is characterised by increased glomerular volume secondary to basement membrane thickening and mesangial enlargement, hyaline deposits and glomerular sclerosis due to mesangial expansion and/or ischaemia. Other histological features may be present such as interstitial fibrosis and tubular atrophy (Figure 8.24).

Approximately 20–50% of patients with diabetes will develop nephropathy. Those who develop diabetes before the age of 15 years are at higher risk. About 35% of T1DM patients will develop nephropathy, although there is evidence of a declining incidence. After about 20 years of diabetes duration in T1DM, the incidence of diabetic nephropathy falls off. The risk of developing diabetic nephropathy varies between individuals and is influenced not only by duration of diabetes but by other factors such as blood pressure, glycaemic control and genetic susceptibility. Nevertheless, diabetic nephropathy is the leading cause of chronic kidney disease (CKD) in the US and other Western societies and is responsible for 30–40% of all end-stage renal disease (ESRD) cases in the US.

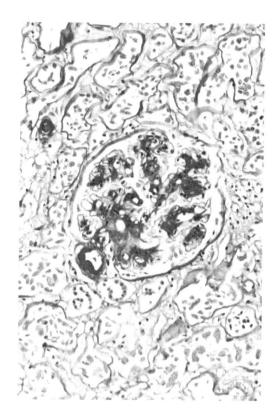

Figure 8.24 Hyalin deposition in the glomerular tuft in a patient with diabetic glomerulopathy. Other characteristic histopathological changes of diabetic nephropathy are an increase in glomerular volume, basement membrane thickening and diffuse mesangial enlargement (often with nodular periodic acid-Schiff-positive lesions). Diabetic nephropathy develops in around 35% of type 1 diabetes mellitus cases and in less than 20% of type 2 diabetes mellitus cases. It is defined as persistent proteinuria (albumin excretion rate >300 mg/day) associated with hypertension and a falling glomerular filtration rate. Established nephropathy is preceded by years of microalbuminuria (albumin excretion rate 30–300 mg/day), which is negative on reagent-strip testing for albumin. Vigorous control of blood pressure and the use of angiotensin-converting enzyme inhibitors have been shown to delay the rate of progression of diabetic nephropathy. Periodic acid-Schiff stain was used.

The severity and incidence of diabetic nephropathy is greater in the Black population and in other ethnic groups. Patients with T1DM and established proteinuria have a greatly increased mortality rate. Because T2DM is much more common globally, the majority of diabetic patients proceeding to end-stage renal failure has this form of diabetes.

The hypertension of diabetic nephropathy appears to be of renal origin and to occur after the onset of microalbuminuria. As proteinuria also reflects widespread vascular damage affecting both small and large vessels, the condition is associated with a poor prognosis unless special strategies are adopted. The causes of death include not only end-stage renal failure, but also myocardial infarction, cardiac failure and cerebrovascular accidents. T2DM patients with nephropathy are more likely to die because of major vascular disease than uraemia.

Peripheral vascular disease, neuropathy and retinopathy are common accompaniments of diabetic nephropathy to the extent that if neuropathy and retinopathy are not present, an alternative cause of the proteinuria should be sought. The sudden development of nephrotic syndrome, a rapid decline in renal function, haematuria and a short duration of T1DM also indicate the need to seek an alternative cause, with the use of renal biopsy, if necessary. If there is a marked discrepancy in size between the kidneys on ultrasound scanning, investigations should be conducted to exclude renal artery stenosis, which is common in diabetes, especially in T2DM with other evidence of vascular disease. Angiotensin-converting enzyme (ACE) inhibitors should be avoided in this situation. Regular monitoring of eGFR and plotting the inverse of serum creatinine against time will give an indication of the rate of progression of nephropathy; however, this may be slowed by vigorous treatment of the associated hypertension, preferably with ACE inhibitors, which have the additional benefit of reducing intraglomerular pressure. Inhibition of the renal-angiotensin-aldosterone system (RAAS) is the key intervention in diabetic nephropathy with landmark trials demonstrating a reduction in the progression of albuminuria in T1DM patients treated with ACE inhibitors. In T2DM, strong trial evidence showed a highly significant benefit from the blockage of the RAAS with angiotensin receptor blockers (ARBs) including a 20% reduction in the composite endpoint of doubling of the serum creatinine, ESRD or death with the use of irbesartan versus placebo in diabetic nephropathy (with similar results with losartan). Dual treatment with an ACE inhibitor and an ARB is contraindicated because of adverse effects. Treatment of hypertension is fundamental to the management of diabetic nephropathy to reduce the associated cardiovascular risk and the risk of progression to advanced

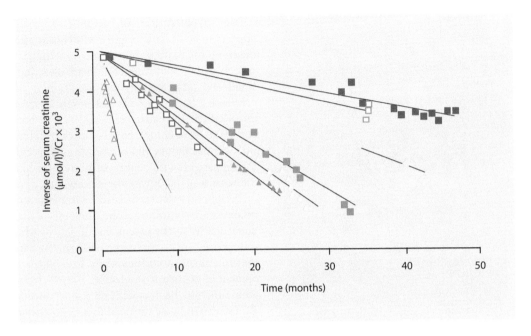

Figure 8.25 Once renal failure has become established in diabetes, there is an inexorable decline in renal function which, if untreated, leads to end-stage renal failure. The decline in renal function is linear when plotted as the inverse of serum creatinine over time. Modern treatment strategies attempt to slow the deterioration of renal function by vigorous antihypertensive regimens. Angiotensin-converting enzyme inhibitors and angiotensin receptor blockers may be especially effective because they reduce intraglomerular pressure and, unless renal failure is advanced, it is still worthwhile to attempt to achieve improved glycaemic control.

renal disease. Guidelines recommend a lowering of blood pressure to less than 130/80 in those with diabetes and albuminuria to achieve optimal renal and cardiovascular protection. Smoking cessation and lipid-lowering therapy are also paramount in this context (Figure 8.25).

There is evidence that establishing strict glycaemic control retards the progression of established nephropathy. The DCCT study in patients with T1DM revealed a significant reduction in the development of moderate and severe albuminuria in the intensively treated arm of the trial. Similar results for an improvement in glycaemic control were also seen in T2DM studies (Action in Diabetes and Vascular Disease: Preterax and Diamicron Modified Release Controlled Evaluation [ADVANCE], VETERANS AFFAIRS DIABETES TRIAL). Importantly, sodium-glucose co-transporter-2 (SGLT2) inhibitors have a significant reno-protective effect in patients with T2DM and are recommended in the American Diabetes Association (ADA) and European Association for the Study of Diabetes (EASD) guidelines for

T2DM patients with diabetic renal disease who need a drug additional to metformin to attain target glycaemic control. In 2021, the US Food and Drug Administration (FDA) approved finerenone (Kerendia), a selective mineralocorticoid receptor antagonist, for the treatment of CKD in patients with diabetes mellitus (DM) based on the findings of the Finerenone in Reducing Kidney Failure and Disease Progression in Diabetic Kidney Disease (FIDELIO-DKD) trial, but treatment with an ACE inhibitor or an ARB take precedence in its management. With declining renal function, insulin requirements fall and, as most sulphonylureas and metformin undergo renal excretion or metabolism, these compounds should not be used in patients with renal failure; in such cases, insulin treatment is preferable, although some agents, such as gliclazide which are cleared predominantly through the liver, may be relatively safe.

With aggressive treatment of hypertension and hyperlipidaemia and improvement of glycaemic control, the need for renal replacement therapy may be delayed for several years. However, late referral of diabetic patients with advanced diabetic nephropathy to a nephrologist should be avoided: referral should be instigated when serum creatinine levels start to rise, and certainly before they reach 300 µmol/l. Renal physicians prefer to see such patients earlier rather than later. Although renal transplantation offers the best method of treatment in suitable patients, haemodialysis is indicated in patients unsuitable for transplantation, while awaiting transplantation or following graft failure. Dialysis may need to be started at lower creatinine levels than in non-diabetic patients because of the tendency to increased fluid retention and volume-dependent hypertension. Vascular access and arterio-venous fistulae failures are additional problems for diabetic patients, as is difficulty achieving blood-glucose control during haemodialysis. However, the prognosis of diabetic patients receiving haemodialysis, although poorer than in non-diabetic subjects, has improved dramatically over the past 20 years.

Long-term survival of diabetic patients with continuous ambulatory peritoneal dialysis (CAPD) is possible. Survival rates may be lower than in non-diabetic patients receiving CAPD. Advantages of CAPD include that vascular access is not required and that good glycaemic control may be achieved by the intraperitoneal route of insulin.

Renal transplantation is the treatment of choice for those <65 years who are free of significant cardiovascular disease, cerebrovascular disease and significant sepsis, and for whom a suitable donor may be found. Survival rates for diabetic patients who receive grafts from living donors are now almost the same as for non-diabetic patients, while results of cadaver transplantation, although less favourable, have improved greatly. Histological changes compatible with diabetic nephropathy can be detected in most transplanted kidneys. Today, many diabetic patients with end-stage renal failure who require a transplant receive both a kidney and a pancreas at the same time.

A major Finnish study of 20,005 patients with T1DM showed that during a follow-up of 35 years, the overall incidence of end-stage renal failure was only 2.2% at 20 years and 7.8% at 30 years after diagnosis. The risk of end-stage renal failure was virtually zero for the first 15 years after diagnosis. These data suggest a greatly improved renal outlook for patients with T1DM, especially for those under age 50. Overall survival has also improved.

DIABETIC NEUROPATHY

Diabetic neuropathy, a common complication of diabetes, is a heterogeneous disorder that encompasses a wide range of abnormalities affecting proximal and distal peripheral sensory and motor nerves as well as the autonomic nervous system (Figure 8.26).

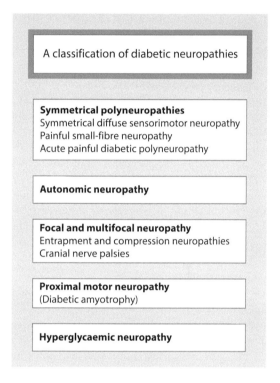

Figure 8.26 Diabetic neuropathy is a common and often disabling complication of diabetes. Distal symmetrical polyneuropathy is the most common form of diabetic neuropathy and can be either sensory or motor and involve small fibres, large fibres or both. Large-fibre neuropathies can involve sensory or motor nerves or both resulting in abnormalities of motor function, vibration perception, position sense and cold-thermal perception with, commonly, a 'glove and stocking' distribution of sensory loss. Small-fibre neuropathy is manifested by pain and paraesthesiae but may develop into a chronic painful neuropathy. Mononeuropathies and entrapment syndromes are common. Proximal motor neuropathies (diabetic amyotrophy) have more complex aetiologies, but are usually associated with great pain and disability. Autonomic neuropathy is rare and leads to a wide variety of symptoms correlating with the affected autonomic nerve damage. After 20 years of diabetes, about 40% of patients will have diabetic neuropathy.

Prevalence

The exact prevalence of diabetic neuropathy is unknown, partly because of difficulties with definition, but it is estimated that as many as 50% of patients with diabetes will have demonstrable evidence of diabetic nerve damage. It is known, however, that the risk of developing neuropathy is directly linked to the duration of diabetes: after 20 years of diabetes, about 40% of patients will have neuropathy. Other significant risk factors for the development of diabetic neuropathy are poor glycaemic control, heavy alcohol use and tall height. In patients attending a diabetic clinic, 25% reported symptoms, 50% were found to have neuropathy using a simple clinical test and almost 90% tested positive with more sophisticated tests. Neuropathy may be present at the time of diagnosis of T2DM, but neurological complications occur equally in T1DM and T2DM. Neuropathy may lead to a significant reduction in quality of life and is a major determinant of foot ulceration and amputation.

Pathogenesis

The pathogenesis of diabetic neuropathy is unknown, but there is no doubt that hyperglycaemia is an important factor. Pathological studies demonstrate axonal degeneration with segmental demyelination and remyelination. Narrowing of the vasa nervorum may also be contributory. Neurophysiological studies show reduced motor and sensory nerve conduction velocities. Abnormalities of the polyol pathway have been invoked as a cause of diabetic neuropathy. In animals, elevated glucose levels in peripheral nerves lead to increased activity of aldose reductase, with consequent increased concentrations of sorbitol and fructose, accompanied by a decrease in the polyol myoinositol. This may lead to reduced membrane sodium–potassium–ATPase activity. It has been postulated that such changes may be reversed by the use of aldose reductase inhibitors. Although these agents have been shown clinically to improve neural conduction velocity, their role in the treatment of diabetic neuropathy remains to be elucidated. Non-enzymatic glycosylation of nerve proteins and lipids resulting in advanced glycation end products (AGEs) that may disrupt neuronal integrity and repair mechanisms and ischaemia caused by increased oxidative stress

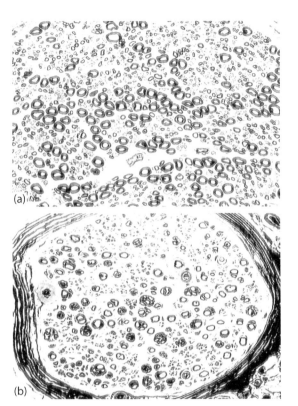

(a)

(b)

Figure 8.27 Transverse semithin sections of resin-embedded sural nerve biopsy specimens stained with thionin and acridine orange. Appearance of a normal nerve (a). Nerve from a patient with diabetic neuropathy shows a loss of myelinated nerve fibres and the presence of regenerative clusters (b). The walls of the endoneural capillaries are thickened. Diabetic neuropathy is a common complication that usually manifests as a sensory, motor or combined symmetrical polyneuropathy. Acute painful neuropathy and diabetic amyotrophy both cause acute pain in the thighs or legs, associated with muscle wasting and weight loss. Painful neuropathy may respond to tricyclic drugs, especially amitriptyline or anticonvulsants, such as gabapentin.

and the production of free radicals may also be significant factors in the development of diabetic neuropathy (Figure 8.27).

Chronic insidious sensory neuropathy

Chronic insidious sensory neuropathy is the most frequently encountered neuropathy in diabetes with paraesthesiae, discomfort, pain, distal sensory loss, loss of vibration sense and reduced or absent tendon reflexes. This type of neuropathy is usually refractory to treatment.

Acute neuropathy

Acute painful neuropathy is relatively uncommon and usually occurs in the context of poor glycaemic control (or a sudden improvement in glycaemic control). Lower limb pain may be particularly severe and accompanied by muscle weakness and wasting. Recovery usually occurs within a year with good control of the diabetes.

Diabetic mononeuropathy

Diabetic mononeuropathies, affecting single nerves or their roots, also occur (Figure 8.28). They are usually of rapid onset and severe in nature, although eventual recovery is the rule in most cases. Such features may point to an acute vascular event as causation rather than chronic metabolic disturbance. Such neuropathies occur mainly in older patients, usually male. When two or more nerve palsies occur within a short time-frame, mononeuritis multiplex must be excluded. Truncal radiculopathies are also encountered, occurring in a dermatomal distribution over the thorax or abdomen (with possible local bulging of the abdominal wall). The acute asymmetrical pain is described as burning or aching and is frequently intensified at night with sensitivity to touch. Cranial nerve lesions are seen relatively frequently. Third-nerve palsies occur most

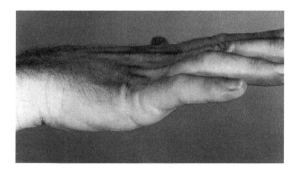

Figure 8.28 This diabetic patient has an ulnar neuropathy. Such entrapment neuropathies are commonly seen in diabetic patients, the most common being carpal tunnel syndrome. It has been postulated that diabetic nerves may be more susceptible to mechanical injury.

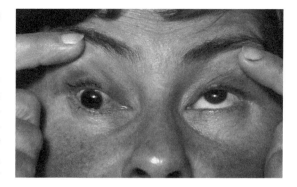

Figure 8.29 Diabetic right-third cranial nerve palsy. The right eye is deviated outwards and downwards, and there is associated ptosis. Pupillary sparing is often encountered. Third-nerve palsy is the most commonly seen cranial neuropathy of diabetes, although fourth-, sixth- and seventh-nerve lesions have also been reported as well as intercostal and phrenic nerve lesions. These lesions usually improve over time.

commonly, although fourth-, sixth- and seventh-nerve lesions are also described (Figure 8.29).

Proximal motor neuropathy

Proximal motor neuropathy (diabetic radiculoplexus neuropathy, femoral neuropathy or diabetic amyotrophy) is a particularly devastating neurological complication of diabetes. It can be identified clinically by certain common features. It primarily affects the elderly and is of gradual or abrupt onset beginning with pain in the thighs and hips or buttocks. Weakness of the proximal muscles of the lower limbs follows. The condition begins unilaterally but often spreads bilaterally and is associated with weight loss and depression. Slow, sometimes incomplete, recovery usually occurs, but may take several months to a year or more. Electrophysiological evaluation reveals a lumbosacral plexopathy, and the condition is now thought to be secondary to a variety of causes that occur more frequently in diabetes, such as chronic inflammatory demyelinating polyneuropathy, monoclonal gammopathy and inflammatory vasculitis. If found to be immune mediated, resolution may be very prompt with immunotherapy. Mononeuropathies must be distinguished from entrapment syndromes. Common entrapment sites in diabetic patients involve median, ulnar, radial, femoral and lateral cutaneous nerves of the thigh. Carpal tunnel syndrome occurs twice as frequently in diabetic patients compared with the normal population.

Diabetic autonomic neuropathy

Damage to the autonomic nervous system, or autonomic neuropathy, is seen in diabetic patients, although the exact prevalence is unknown, reported prevalence rates in studies vary widely (Figure 8.30). Tests of autonomic nerve function often reveal abnormalities in patients with no symptoms of autonomic dysfunction. These tests include the heart-rate response to the Valsalva manoeuvre, to deep breathing and to moving from the supine to the erect posture, and the blood pressure response to sustained handgrip and standing up. Cardiovascular tests are relatively simple to perform, but evaluating the autonomic control of other systems, such as the gastrointestinal tract and micturition, is much more complex.

Diabetic autonomic neuropathy produces dysfunction in the cardiovascular system, the gastrointestinal system, the genitourinary system and the sweat glands. This results in a wide spectrum of autonomic symptoms, including male impotence, postural hypotension, sinus arrhythmia, nocturnal diarrhoea, faecal incontinence, nausea and vomiting, gustatory sweating, heavy sweating of the face, neck and trunk, diminished or absent sweating in the feet, a feeling of incomplete bladder emptying and loss of awareness of acute hypoglycaemia, plus many other rarer manifestations of autonomic dysfunction. Gastric atony (diabetic gastroparesis), especially when associated with vomiting, results in loss of glycaemic control in insulin-treated subjects (Figure 8.31). Bladder enlargement with defective micturition is also reported. Resting tachycardia is a common sign. Many studies have

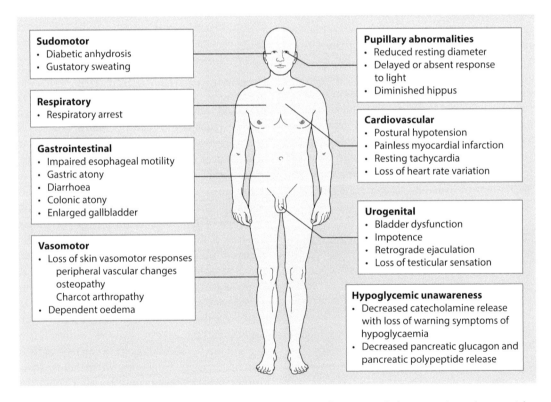

Sudomotor
• Diabetic anhydrosis
• Gustatory sweating

Respiratory
• Respiratory arrest

Gastrointestinal
• Impaired esophageal motility
• Gastric atony
• Diarrhoea
• Colonic atony
• Enlarged gallbladder

Vasomotor
• Loss of skin vasomotor responses
  peripheral vascular changes
  osteopathy
  Charcot arthropathy
• Dependent oedema

Pupillary abnormalities
• Reduced resting diameter
• Delayed or absent response to light
• Diminished hippus

Cardiovascular
• Postural hypotension
• Painless myocardial infarction
• Resting tachycardia
• Loss of heart rate variation

Urogenital
• Bladder dysfunction
• Impotence
• Retrograde ejaculation
• Loss of testicular sensation

Hypoglycemic unawareness
• Decreased catecholamine release with loss of warning symptoms of hypoglycaemia
• Decreased pancreatic glucagon and pancreatic polypeptide release

Figure 8.30 Clinical features of diabetic autonomic neuropathy. Many diabetic patients have evidence of autonomic dysfunction, but very few have autonomic symptoms. The most prominent symptom is postural hypotension. Erectile dysfunction, common in diabetic men, is not always due to autonomic neuropathy. Late manifestations other than postural hypotension include gustatory sweating, diabetic diarrhoea, gastric atony and reduced awareness of hypoglycaemia. Symptomatic autonomic neuropathy may be associated with a poor prognosis.

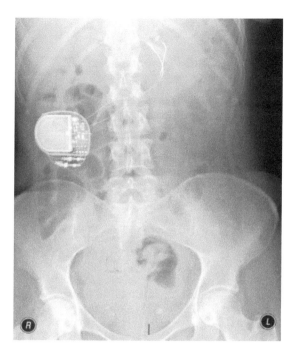

Figure 8.31 Intractable vomiting due to diabetic gastroparesis is notoriously difficult to treat. This patient was successfully treated by the surgical implantation of the Enterra™ Gastric Neurostimulator (GES) system (Medtronic Inc, Minneapolis, US). This novel experimental approach may prove to be an effective treatment strategy in such rare but difficult-to-treat patients.

suggested that once symptomatic autonomic neuropathy is present, the life prognosis for the patient is significantly diminished.

Treatment of diabetic neuropathy

Improving glycaemic control has been shown to slow the progression of neuropathy. Various agents, other than simple analgesics and NSAIDs, have been used to diminish the distressing discomfort associated with painful diabetic neuropathies. Tricyclic antidepressants, such as amitriptyline, which have a central action that modifies pain perception, and serotonin-noradrenaline (norepinephrine) reuptake inhibitors, such as duloxetine and venlafaxine, are recommended first-line agents for the treatment of pain when simple agents are ineffective. Anticonvulsants, such as gabapentin, sodium valproate and pregabalin, are useful in the treatment of painful neuropathy as first- or second-line agents. It

may be necessary, when the drugs mentioned here fail, to deliver acceptable pain relief (considered in this context to be a 50% reduction in pain levels) to exhibit opioid drugs such as tramadol, but caution must be exercised to avoid the risk of addiction. Localised transdermal lignocaine (lidocaine) has also been shown to be effective.

Non-pharmacological therapies include nerve stimulation therapies and electrical spinal-cord stimulation. It is, however, recognised that despite pharmacological treatment, many patients continue to experience pain or discomfort, and treatment may be considered successful in patients who experience a moderate decrease in pain or improved function. Depletion of axonal neuropeptide substance P with capsaicin extracted from chilli peppers may help in some patients with C-fibre pain. The combination of erythromycin and metoclopramide is recommended for the treatment of gastroparesis.

MAJOR VASCULAR DISEASE

Although microvascular disease is a major concern in diabetic patients, it should be emphasised that most patients with long-term T1DM and most patients with T2DM will die because of cardiovascular disease. Diabetic patients have an excess mortality, owing to coronary artery disease, compared with the non-diabetic control population. Although death rates from coronary heart disease have fallen in the US, this has not been observed in the diabetic population. Additionally, a three-fold risk of death from cardiovascular disease was seen in men with diabetes compared to non-diabetic men in the Multiple Risk Factor Intervention Trial (MRFIT). Excess cardiovascular mortality also occurs in females. There is also an increased mortality due to peripheral vascular disease and stroke. Diabetes is an independent risk factor for stroke, especially in a younger population. Mechanisms for vasculopathy in diabetes include vascular endothelial dysfunction, increased arterial stiffness and systemic inflammation. Diabetic patients account for about 60% of all non-traumatic lower-limb amputations in the US. Atheromatous lesions in diabetic patients are histologically identical to those in the non-diabetic population, but are more severe and widespread. Coronary artery disease may progress more quickly and, hence, present at a younger age (Figures 8.32–8.37).

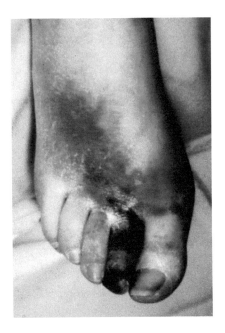

Figure 8.32 Distal gangrene in a diabetic ischaemic foot (dorsal view).

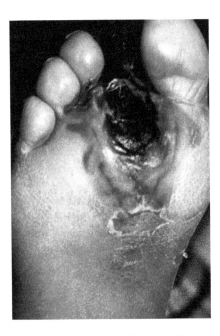

Figure 8.33 Plantar view of the same foot as in Figure 8.32 shows the common diabetic complications of ischaemia and neuropathy, both of which may lead to ulceration. The ischaemic foot is cold, pulseless and subject to rest pain, ulceration and gangrene (shown here). Ischaemic ulceration usually affects the margins of the foot and may be amenable to angioplasty or reconstructive arterial surgery.

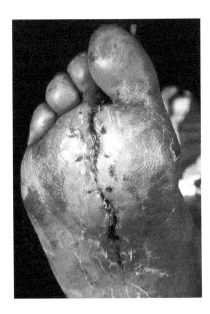

Figure 8.34 The same foot as in Figures 8.32 and 8.33 after amputation of the second toe. A good result has been obtained. However, a large proportion of diabetic patients with critical ischaemia or gangrene of the lower limbs undergo major amputation. Thus, the importance of adequate screening and preventive measures to avoid these operations cannot be overemphasised.

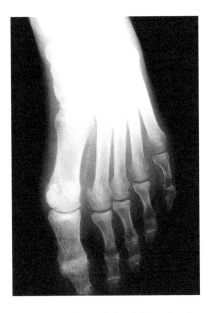

Figure 8.35 Digital arterial calcification in a diabetic foot. Peripheral vascular disease is a particularly common vascular complication of diabetes and about half of all lower limb amputations involve diabetic patients.

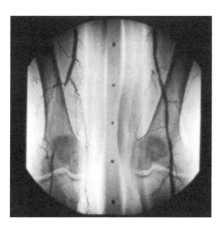

Figure 8.36 Angiogram showing occlusion of the right popliteal artery at the adductor canal in a diabetic patient with peripheral vascular disease (left). There are many collateral vessels and the artery reconstitutes distally below the knee. The opposite side (right), which is normal, is shown for comparison.

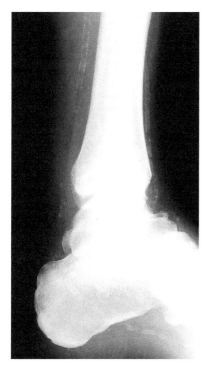

Figure 8.37 Calcification accompanying medial sclerosis of the distal lower limb arteries. In diabetes, the distal blood vessels are often affected by both atheroma and medial sclerosis with calcification. This must be borne in mind if reconstructive vascular surgery or percutaneous transluminal balloon angioplasty is contemplated for symptomatic peripheral vascular disease. The initial success rate with angioplasty is reduced in diabetic patients.

Hyperglycaemia during acute coronary syndrome is associated with a worse outcome. The Diabetes Mellitus Insulin Glucose infusion in Acute Myocardial Infarction (DIGAMI) study demonstrated a 11% reduction in mortality at 1 year in patients treated intensively with insulin at the time of a myocardial infarction and for a minimum of 3 months thereafter. Diabetic patients with an acute STEMI should be treated promptly with revascularisation with fibrinolysis and primary percutaneous coronary intervention (PCI). Nevertheless, even if reperfusion is achieved, diabetic patients have a higher mortality than non-diabetic subjects, particularly those with a recurrent myocardial infarction. Diabetes may also cause a specific cardiomyopathy in the absence of coronary artery disease.

Although risk factors for macrovascular disease that pertain to the general population are also relevant to diabetic patients, haemostatic abnormalities (for example, decreased fibrinolysis or increased fibrinogen levels), hypertension and hyperlipidaemia are particularly important in the latter. Hyperinsulinaemia and insulin resistance are considered to be significant risk factors for the development of atherosclerosis.

HYPERTENSION

Hypertension is a major risk factor in the development of diabetic complications, both macrovascular and microvascular. Therefore, its detection and treatment are of vital importance in overall diabetic management. Hypertension is common in diabetes: study prevalence rates vary, but it affects more than 50% of patients with T2DM. The prevalence rate is less in patients with T1DM, where it is particularly associated with incipient and established nephropathy. It is a major risk factor for stroke and coronary artery disease, but also aggravates nephropathy and retinopathy. Blood pressure starts to rise when microalbuminuria develops, and the close link between hypertension and nephropathy may be explained by genetic factors leading to an increased susceptibility to develop, both associated with increased sodium–lithium counter-transport activity in red blood cells. It is now thought that the common link between obesity, diabetes, hyperlipidaemia and hypertension in T2DM is insulin resistance and associated hyperinsulinaemia, either inherited or perhaps acquired through malnutrition in early life. Occasionally, hypertension is associated with renal artery stenosis, and this should be investigated, and ACE inhibitors and ARBs avoided, when this clinical suspicion arises.

The ADA guidelines for the treatment of hypertension in diabetes patients recommend initiation of therapy if blood pressure is 140/90 or greater with a target blood pressure of less than 140/90 (lower in high-risk patients). Other guidelines recommend a lower target blood pressure e.g. less than 130/80. It has been suggested that targets for blood pressure lowering should be lower than for the non-diabetic population because of the major adverse effect of hypertension in this group. However, caution is advised as the Action to Control Cardiovascular Risk in Diabetes (ACCORD) blood pressure trial of lowering systolic blood pressure (SBP) to a target of 120 mm Hg versus 140 mm Hg showed no difference in primary cardiovascular outcomes between groups, but an increased incidence of adverse events in the lower SBP group. The Blood Pressure Control Study incorporated into the UKPDS demonstrated that a tight blood pressure control policy achieving a mean blood pressure of 144/82 gave a reduced risk for any diabetes-related endpoint, diabetes-related death, stroke, microvascular disease, heart failure and progression of retinopathy. It also demonstrated that in many patients, combination therapy was necessary to achieve this level of blood pressure control. However, effective blood pressure reduction is likely to be more achievable than effective blood glucose control.

ACE inhibitors (captopril, enalapril, lisinopril, fosinopril, ramipril, etc.) and ARBs (candesartan, irbesartan, olmesartan, azilsartan, losartan, etc.) are the first-line choice to treat diabetic hypertension, as not only are they effective, but they also delay the progression of diabetic retinopathy and diabetic nephropathy (perhaps in the latter by reducing intraglomerular pressure). The effect of ramipril in reducing the rates of death, myocardial infarction and stroke in a broad range of high-risk patients, about 40% of whom had diabetes, was demonstrated in the Heart Outcomes Prevention Evaluation (HOPE) study. Second-line agents recommended for the treatment of diabetic hypertension (or first-line when ACE inhibitors and ARBs cannot be tolerated or are contraindicated) include thiazide-like diuretics (indapamide, chlorthalidone) and calcium channel blockers (amlodipine, felodipine, isradipine).

THE DIABETIC FOOT

Foot ulceration represents a common, but potentially serious, complication of diabetes. The estimated prevalence of diabetic foot ulcers is 13% in North America and 6.4% globally. There is a 2–5% annual incidence of foot ulceration or necrosis and 1% may end up with an amputation. Diabetic foot lesions are responsible for more hospital admissions than any other complication of diabetes. Diabetic patients with foot ulceration are at a higher risk of death than those without foot ulcers. The associated healthcare costs are enormous. In 2014, it was estimated that diabetic foot ulceration in the US cost $9–13 billion USD in excess of costs related to diabetes generally. In 2018, a UK study showed that diabetic foot ulceration cost £7800 per healed ulcer and £16,900 per amputation. The tragedy of this, from both a patient and economic perspective, is that such morbidity and costs result from lesions that are potentially preventable by the institution of, and compliance with, diabetic foot care policies.

The main antecedents of diabetic foot ulceration are poor glycaemic control, callus formation, neuropathy, medium- and small-vessel peripheral vascular disease, improper foot care, ill-fitting footwear, dry skin and abnormal foot biomechanics (Figure 8.38). These factors are frequently compounded by bacterial infection. The range of organisms associated with diabetic foot ulceration is diverse but *Staphylococcus aureus, Pseudomonas*

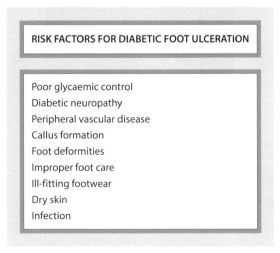

RISK FACTORS FOR DIABETIC FOOT ULCERATION

Poor glycaemic control
Diabetic neuropathy
Peripheral vascular disease
Callus formation
Foot deformities
Improper foot care
Ill-fitting footwear
Dry skin
Infection

Figure 8.38 Risk factors for diabetic foot ulceration.

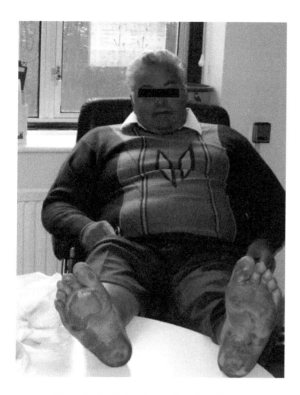

Figure 8.39 This diabetic patient had known diabetic neuropathy and had been repeatedly given foot care advice in his diabetes centre. Despite this, he walked over a hot surface in a Mediterranean country in a summer month. By the time he realised that there was a problem, he had sustained extensive burn injuries to both feet, requiring urgent medical attention.

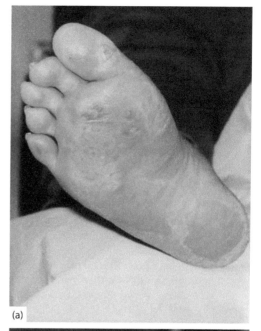

(a)

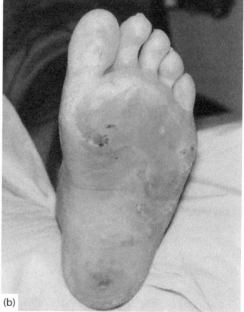

(b)

Figure 8.40 In spite of his diabetes and neuropathy, and with good care from the podiatrist, this patient's burns healed remarkably quickly, fortunately with no adverse sequelae.

and *Escherichia coli* species predominate followed by *Proteus, Klebsiella* and *Enterococcus. Bacteroides* species occur rarely. Neuropathy is thought to be the main causative factor in the development of ulcers with trauma occurring as a result of loss of pain sensation. Minimal trauma, such as a foreign body in the shoes, ill-fitting shoes or walking barefoot on a hot surface, may lead to devastating effects (see Figures 8.39 and 8.40). Non-enzymatic glycosylation of skin and connective tissue, together with reduced collagen production, may result in altered biomechanics in the diabetic foot. Excessive pressure loading on the sole, especially over the metatarsal heads and heels, predisposes to the formation of calluses, which can break down and lead to ulceration. Indeed, the callus is an important predictor of ulceration. Such excess pressure is generated by motor-nerve damage, altering the posture of the foot, limited joint mobility and local deformities including Charcot arthropathy (Figure 8.41). Autonomic nerve damage leads to reduced sweating and a dry skin which may crack or split more easily, allowing the ingress of infection. Atherosclerotic disease of

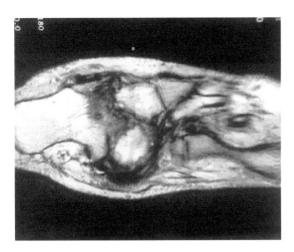

Figure 8.41 Magnetic resonance image of a diabetic foot showing disorganisation of the talocalcaneonavicular joint with erosions of the articular surface. Such appearances in a diabetic patient are typical of a Charcot joint.

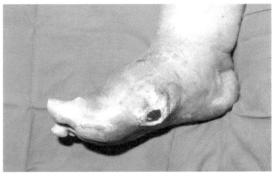

Figure 8.42 This neuropathic ulcer on the medial aspect of the foot in a diabetic patient shows the characteristic punched-out appearance on heavily calloused skin. The neuropathic foot is numb, warm and dry with palpable pulses. Charcot arthropathy complicates the neuropathic foot and presents with warmth, swelling and redness (shown here). Ulceration occurs at areas of high pressure in the deformed foot, especially over the metatarsal heads. Minor trauma, such as ill-fitting or new shoes, or the presence of a small undetected object in the shoe can result in serious foot ulceration. Treatment is by bedrest, debridement and appropriate antibiotics to treat secondary infection. Special shoes and plaster casts (to allow mobility while taking pressure off the ulcer) are also useful.

the peripheral vessels, especially the small vessels, is common in diabetic patients and is an important predisposing factor in most cases of diabetic foot ulceration. Ulcers attributable purely to ischaemia are relatively rare and, as neuropathy usually co-exists, such ulcers are described as neuroischaemic as opposed to the more common neuropathic ulcers where neuropathy is the critical antecedent factor. When ulcers are infected, they exhibit local signs of inflammation such as erythema, warmth and tenderness, although such signs might be unimpressive despite definite infection. Deep-seated infection and osteomyelitis are important to diagnose. If bone can be felt when probing an ulcer, osteomyelitis can be assumed. Deep infection is suggested by the presence of deep sinuses, a foul discharge and crepitus on palpating the foot (Figures 8.38–8.40, 8.42–49).

It follows from the previous discussion that risk factors for the development of diabetic foot ulcers include the presence of neuropathy (and other microvascular complications), peripheral vascular disease, previous amputation and foot deformity, together with previous foot ulceration, poor foot care advice and advanced age.

The management of diabetic foot ulceration is complicated and requires great expertise and experience, particularly because many approaches to treatment are not evidence based. A multidisciplinary approach is

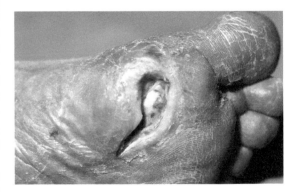

Figure 8.43 A deeply penetrating diabetic neuropathic ulcer over the metatarsal head caused by a foreign body. Foot education, especially in those patients with documented neuropathy, is essential for preventing such lesions and should be undertaken by chiropodists, diabetic specialist nurses and diabetic physicians. Diabetic patients should not put their feet in front of fires or on radiators. Their feet should also be regularly inspected for early ulceration and their shoes carefully checked for foreign objects before being worn.

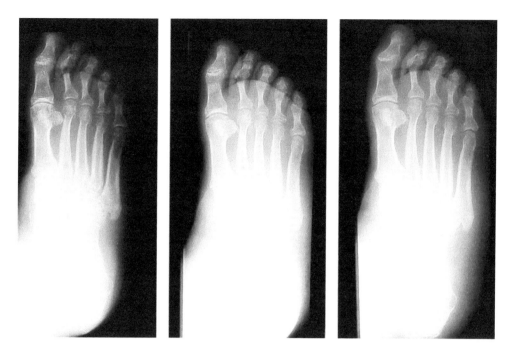

Figure 8.44 Three radiographs of the same neuropathic foot taken 1 month apart. Progressive damage to the foot has led to complete disorganisation of the midtarsal joints without osteoporosis. These are typical appearances of a Charcot joint.

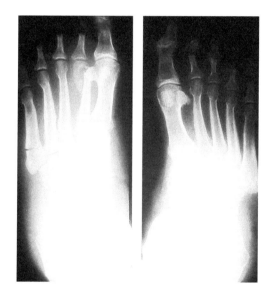

Figure 8.45 Radiographs of the feet of a diabetic patient showing a neuropathic ulcer over the metatarsal heads of the left foot. Destruction of the left second metatarsal head and associated soft-tissue swelling are secondary to osteomyelitis, complicating the ulcer. A fracture on the base of the fifth metatarsal is also present. The right foot shows Charcot disorganisation of the midtarsal joints.

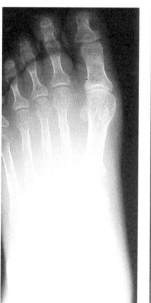
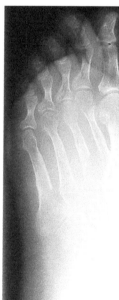

Figure 8.46 Osteomyelitis in the diabetic foot with destruction of the base of the third metatarsal (right) and a periosteal reaction in the shafts of the adjacent metatarsals accompanied by osteoporosis.

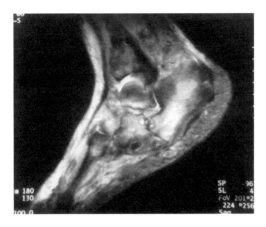

Figure 8.47 Sagittal magnetic resonance image of the hind foot of a diabetic patient showing marrow oedema of the calcaneus consistent with acute osteomyelitis. There is also fluid deep to the plantar fascia, consistent with cellulitis. An ankle effusion is also present.

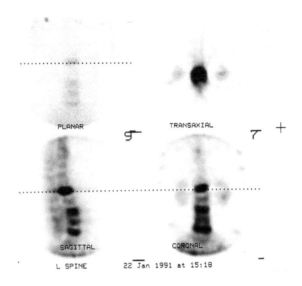

Figure 8.49 Bone scan showing osteoporotic vertebral collapse in a patient with type 1 diabetes mellitus, which has been associated with a generalised reduction in bone density (diabetic osteopaenia). It is probably more common in those patients exhibiting poor metabolic control and is due to reduced bone formation rather than increased resorption. A slightly increased risk of susceptibility to fracture results from this abnormality.

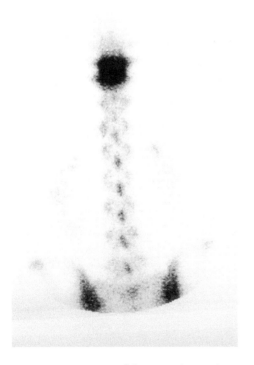

Figure 8.48 Bone scan of the spine (posterior view) in a poorly controlled type 2 diabetes mellitus patient shows the florid increase in activity in adjacent vertebrae typical of osteomyelitis.

warranted involving, as necessary, diabetologists, podiatrists, orthopaedic surgeons, vascular surgeons, microbiologists, primary-care physicians, nurses and orthotists. Debridement and removal of slough and necrotic eschar is vital to promote healing. Surgical debridement may occasionally be necessary for an extensive lesion; however, aggressive debridement should be postponed where severe ischaemia is present or suspected until vascular assessment has been undertaken. For plantar ulcers, off-loading is an important part of treatment (Figure 8.50). Relief of pressure is a basic principle of management of all neuropathic ulcers. The most effective method of off-loading is the use of a non-removable total-contact cast (TCC) made of plastic or fibreglass materials (Figure 8.51). For those who cannot tolerate TCCs, removable casts may also be used. Therapeutic shoes, customised insoles and the use of felted foam are alternatives. Ulcers heal more quickly in a moist environment. Dressings should be absorbent enough to remove excess wound exudation, should maintain a moist environment and be impermeable to microorganisms. Infection must be treated when present,

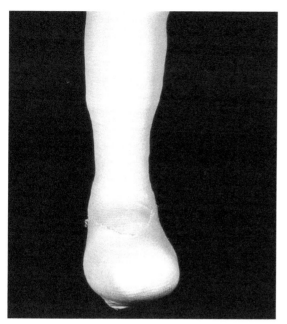

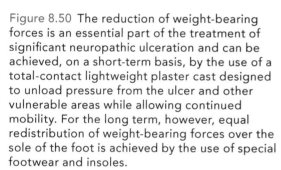

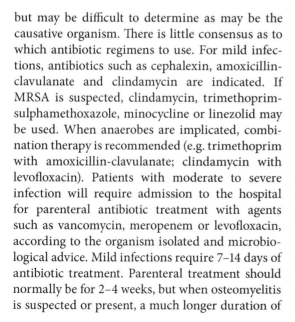

Figure 8.50 The reduction of weight-bearing forces is an essential part of the treatment of significant neuropathic ulceration and can be achieved, on a short-term basis, by the use of a total-contact lightweight plaster cast designed to unload pressure from the ulcer and other vulnerable areas while allowing continued mobility. For the long term, however, equal redistribution of weight-bearing forces over the sole of the foot is achieved by the use of special footwear and insoles.

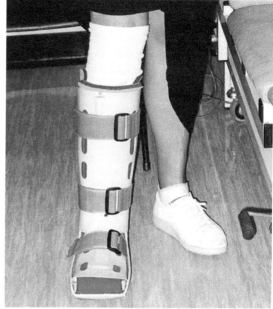

Figure 8.51 Off-loading pressure from diabetic foot ulcers is essential to allow healing. Total contact plaster casts may be used, but are not free from problems. A more recent alternative is the Aircast Pneumatic Walker with a Diabetic Conversion Kit. It is a lightweight removable plastic brace lined with inflatable chambers to promote off-loading. Experience to-date has shown that such a boot greatly increases the immediate off-loading capacity of the diabetic foot clinic.

but may be difficult to determine as may be the causative organism. There is little consensus as to which antibiotic regimens to use. For mild infections, antibiotics such as cephalexin, amoxicillin-clavulanate and clindamycin are indicated. If MRSA is suspected, clindamycin, trimethoprim-sulphamethoxazole, minocycline or linezolid may be used. When anaerobes are implicated, combination therapy is recommended (e.g. trimethoprim with amoxicillin-clavulanate; clindamycin with levofloxacin). Patients with moderate to severe infection will require admission to the hospital for parenteral antibiotic treatment with agents such as vancomycin, meropenem or levofloxacin, according to the organism isolated and microbiological advice. Mild infections require 7–14 days of antibiotic treatment. Parenteral treatment should normally be for 2–4 weeks, but when osteomyelitis is suspected or present, a much longer duration of

antibiotic treatment is necessary, usually of at least 6 weeks. It should be emphasised, however, that the duration of treatment has to be individualised. Routine radiography has a role to play in revealing the presence of gas or evidence of osteomyelitis. It often reveals calcification of the small vessels of the foot. Osteomyelitis can be confirmed by alternative imaging techniques such as magnetic resonance imaging (MRI) or white-cell scanning (Figures 8.46–8.48). In all cases, a vascular assessment should be made and amputation may be necessary if there is extensive gangrene or spreading necrosis in a toxic patient. Revascularisation may be possible for neuroischaemic ulcers.

Bioengineered skin substitutes, either cell-containing (Apligraf, Dermagraft, Hyalograft, Trancell) or acellular (OASIS, GRAFTJACKET), show promise as an adjunct therapy for non-infected diabetic foot ulcers and have been shown

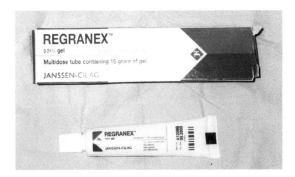

Figure 8.52 A topical preparation of becaplermin (Regranex◆) has been recently introduced as an adjunct in the treatment of full-thickness, neuropathic, diabetic foot ulcers. Becaplermin is a recombinant human platelet-derived growth factor. Experience to-date with this product is limited and it is very expensive. Accurate cost–benefit analyses are awaited.

to shorten healing time and to produce a significantly greater proportion of healed ulcers. The platelet-derived growth factor (PDGF-beta), becaplermin (Regranex), a topical agent used as a once-daily gel in conjunction with debridement, has been shown to improve healing of small low-grade ulcers, but the FDA has issued a warning of an increased risk of cancer with excessive use (Figure 8.52). Hyperbaric oxygen has been shown to accelerate the rate of healing and increase the number of wounds completely healed. Studies have attested to the potential benefit of negative-pressure wound therapy in the treatment of diabetic foot ulcers. Debridement with maggots is simple and effective for cleaning chronic wounds and initiating granulation. None of these techniques has become an accepted standard therapy for the treatment of diabetic foot ulcers, and further assessments of efficacy and cost-effectiveness are required.

The assessment of foot ulcer risk, the dissemination of good foot care advice and early and urgent treatment of established ulceration are the mainstays of the prevention of amputation secondary to diabetic foot ulcers. Comprehensive screening and treatment programmes have been shown to reduce the risk of amputation. Preventative podiatric care should be given to all patients at risk. Simple measures, such as the debridement of callus and the fitting of appropriate shoes, often with the help of

an orthotist, may be all that is necessary to prevent one of the most devastating and feared complications of diabetes: amputation.

ERECTILE DYSFUNCTION IN DIABETES

Erectile dysfunction (ED) is common in diabetes. The reported prevalence in one study was 37.5% in T1DM, 66.3% in T2DM and 57.7% overall, making it one of the most common complications of diabetes (although figures vary). It is now recognised that ED represents a vascular complication of diabetes. Cardiovascular disease increases the risk of ED, but ED itself is probably a risk factor for cardiovascular disease. Certainly, studies have shown an association between ED and most of the cardiovascular risk factors, including smoking, hypertension, hyperlipidaemia, metabolic syndrome and depression. ED in diabetes is most likely a result of a defect in nitric oxide-mediated cavernosal smooth muscle relaxation as a consequence of autonomic nerve damage and endothelial dysfunction. Large vessel disease, advanced age, hypertension, concomitant drug therapy, long duration of diabetes and psychological factors may also contribute. Furthermore, men with diabetes may be at increased risk of having low serum testosterone levels which, together with other factors, may decrease sexual drive. It is important to recognise that diabetic women also are at risk of sexual dysfunction (problems with desire, arousal, lubrication, dyspareunia and orgasm).

Today, male diabetic patients with ED are much more likely to seek advice and treatment. Every opportunity for them to so do should be made available and routine enquiry into sexual function, especially in older patients, may well be appropriate. Few investigations are needed. Measuring serum testosterone is indicated if sex drive is reduced. Other endocrine testing should only be undertaken in the rare situation when a clinical suspicion of hypogonadism exists. A detailed history should be taken to define the precise problem with sexual function.

If a diabetic male with ED wishes treatment for the condition, he should be offered an oral agent as a first-line therapy, assuming there is no contraindication. It is fruitless to try and determine whether the ED has a psychogenic component.

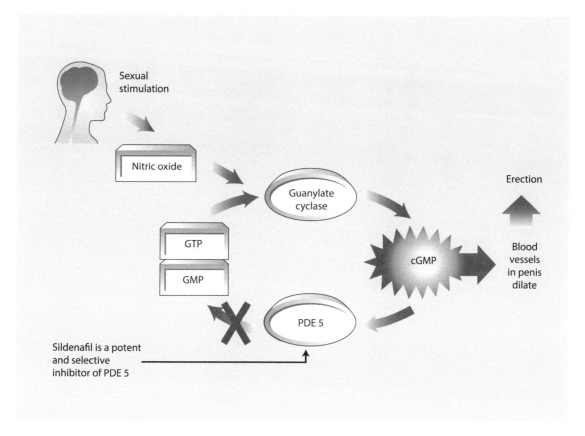

Figure 8.53 Oral treatment of erectile dysfunction with sildenafil is effective in about 60% of patients with diabetes. Sildenafil selectively inhibits phosphodiesterase type 5 (PDE 5), thereby increasing levels of cyclic GMP within the corpora cavernosa. This enhances the natural erectile response to sexual stimulation.

Phosphodiesterase inhibitors (PDE5 inhibitors), such as sildenafil (Viagra®), vardenafil (Levitra/Staxyn), tadalafil (Cialis) and avanafil (Stendra), are the agents of choice (Figure 8.53). Inhibition of this enzyme diminishes the breakdown of nitric oxide via the second messenger cGMP. PDE5 inhibitors only work in the presence of sexual stimulation and have no effect on libido. Recommended doses should be taken 30 minutes to 4 hours before planned sexual activity, depending on the agent used. The most common side effects are headaches, dyspepsia, flushing, nasal congestion and nasopharyngitis. Priapism is a rare complication and calls for immediate medical attention to avoid permanent damage to the penis. PDE5 inhibitors are not associated with an increased risk of cardiovascular events, although the resultant sexual activity may be. Treatment

with nitrates is an absolute contraindication to the use of PDE5 inhibitors, as the combination may produce profound hypotension. Temporary visual changes have been reported. The success rate for PDE5 inhibitors for the treatment of ED in diabetic men is of the order of 50–60%. If one agent is ineffective, a trial of an alternative PDE5 inhibitor is warranted. Once-daily administration of low-dose tadalafil has been licensed by the FDA. With some agents, efficacy may persist for up to 36 hours after administration. Apomorphine, a centrally acting inducer of erections, has been suggested as an alternative to phosphodiesterase inhibitors, but current opinion is that it is of limited benefit.

In those failing to respond to oral agents, erection may be induced by the intracavernosal injection of alprostadil (prostaglandin E1), papaverine and phentolamine, either alone or in combination.

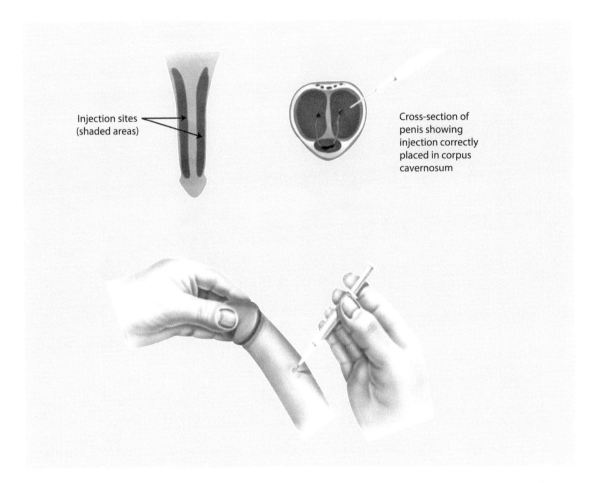

Injection sites
(shaded areas)

Cross-section of
penis showing
injection correctly
placed in corpus
cavernosum

Figure 8.54 Erectile dysfunction in diabetes may be treated by self-injection of the vasoactive drug alprostadil (Caverject, Pharmacia, Peapack, NJ, US) prostaglandin E1 into the corpus cavernosum of the penis. The resultant smooth muscle relaxation allows increased blood flow into the penis, and penile erection will occur whether or not sexual stimulation is present.

However, long-term discontinuation rates are high, penile pain is a relatively common side effect of such therapy and patients must be warned of the much more serious complication of priapism. An alternative mode of delivery of alprostadil is by the transurethral routine using a slender applicator to deposit a pellet containing alprostadil in polyethylene glycol. Such therapy, marketed as Medicated Urethral System for Erection (MUSE), has been successful in about 65% of diabetic men, although often associated with penile pain. Long-term usage rates are not high and some men may actually prefer to inject intracavernosally. Patients with low serum testosterone levels may benefit from replacement therapy (Figures 8.54, 8.55).

Devices which produce a passive penile tumescence by applying a vacuum via a hand or battery operated pump are available (Figure 8.56). Penile engorgement is maintained using a rubber constriction ring at the base of the penis. Although rigidity sufficient for vaginal penetration may be induced in most patients, the quality of erection may not be as good as that achieved by pharmacological methods and many couples may not find such a technique acceptable for a variety of reasons. For those who have failed to respond to the approaches mentioned here, and with careful selection and counselling, the surgical implantation of a penile prosthesis can be a successful treatment for erectile failure

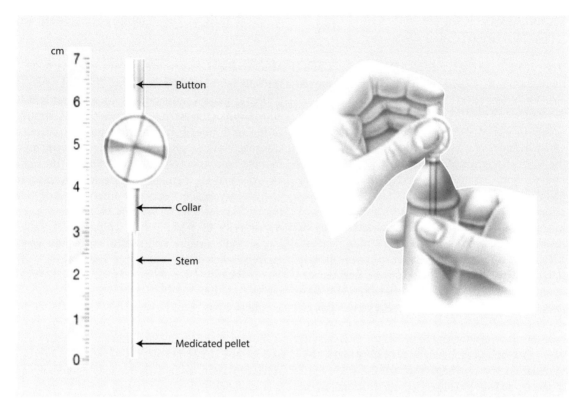

Figure 8.55 An alternative method of administering alprostadil is by transurethral application of a narrow (1.4 mm) pellet of synthetic prostaglandin E1 directly into the male urethra. Although this removes the need to inject alprostadil, there is still an incidence of penile pain, and controversy exists as to the efficacy of this procedure.

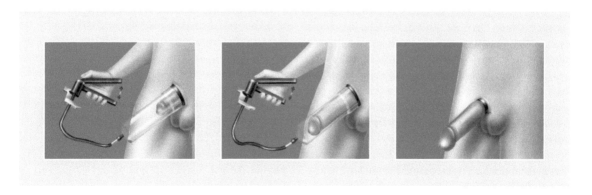

Figure 8.56 A vacuum system for management of diabetic impotence. Placing the cylinder over the penis and creating a vacuum with the pump produces an erection which can be maintained by placing constrictor rings over the base of the penis. Studies have shown that many patients prefer this non-invasive technique to other, more invasive, methods.

NON-ALCOHOLIC STEATOHEPATOSIS

Non-alcoholic fatty liver disease (NAFLD) is a common finding in T2DM (with an estimated prevalence of 70% in obese diabetic adults) and is related to obesity and insulin resistance. It less frequently occurs in T1DM. NAFLD is an overarching term which includes simple hepatic steatosis (excess fat in the form of triglycerides in liver cells, NAFL) and non-alcoholic steatohepatitis (NASH). The main histological finding in NAFL is, thus, excess triglycerides in hepatic cells, while NASH is characterised histologically by steatosis, hepatic cell injury in the form of ballooning and lobular inflammation. Patients with NASH may progress to hepatic fibrosis (cirrhosis), end-stage liver disease and hepatic carcinoma. In one study, 35% of cases of NASH progressed to liver fibrosis. However, the cause of death in patients with NAFLD is more likely to be cardiovascular than hepatic, and some authorities consider NAFLD to be an independent risk factor for cardiovascular disease. NAFLD is the most common cause of abnormal liver blood results among adults in the US. It is particularly common in those with combined diabetes and obesity: in a group of severely obese patients with diabetes, 100% were found to have mild steatosis, 50% had NASH and 19% had cirrhosis. The pathogenesis of NAFLD in diabetes is complex. Insulin resistance seems to be the most reproducible causative factor in the development of NAFLD and this condition is increasingly viewed as part of the spectrum of the metabolic syndrome.

The pathogenesis of NAFLD is complex and not yet fully understood. An incestuous relationship exists between NAFLD and T2DM. The accumulation of hepatic fat may occur as a consequence of dietary fat intake, obesity and insulin resistance, with insulin resistance playing a key role. Deposition of lipid in hepatocytes comes from triacylglycerols derived from free fatty acids (FFAs), *de novo* lipogenesis and diet. Diabetes-related hyperinsulinaemia stimulates lipogenesis with a resultant increase in delivery of FFAs to the liver. Excess stored fat leads to abnormal lipid peroxidation and release of pro-inflammatory cytokines and other factors, which results in liver damage. Other proposed aetiological factors include hyperglycaemia-related glucotoxicity, glucagon resistance, environmental and genetic factors and dysregulation of the gut microbiome. Malaise and a sensation of fullness or discomfort in the right hypochondrium are recognised symptoms when symptoms exist, and hepatomegaly is the only consistent physical sign. Mild to moderate elevation of liver enzymes is often the only laboratory abnormality. The evaluation of patients includes ultrasonography to detect NASH and fibrosis. The ADA guidelines for risk stratification recommend the use of vibration controlled transient elastography (VCTE, Fibroscan) and non-invasive biomarkers. NAFLD is defined by the presence of 5% or greater of hepatic steatosis by imaging or histology in the absence of other causes of liver injury. Various scoring systems are in use to assess the severity of NAFLD (e.g. NFS, BARD). Liver biopsy and histology are the ultimate techniques to quantify steatosis, inflammation and fibrosis.

No entirely satisfactory treatment for NAFLD has been found. Lifestyle intervention to promote weight loss has been shown to be effective in reducing steatosis and inflammation. Fibrosis regression is more difficult to achieve. Bariatric surgery and endoscopic bariatric techniques may also be considered. Therapeutic agents that have been shown to be beneficial include metformin, SGLT2 inhibitors and the thiazolidinedione pioglitazone. Glucagon-like peptide-1 (GLP-1) and gastric inhibitory polypeptide (GIP) receptor agonists have been studied in NAFLD and the dual GLP-1 and GIP agonist tirzepatide shows promise in this area.

THE SKIN IN DIABETES

A variety of disorders of the skin occur in patients with DM. Some of these conditions are associated with endocrine or metabolic disorders that may themselves cause diabetes (Figure 8.57).

Acanthosis nigricans

This skin manifestation is often missed on examination, but is nevertheless fairly frequently encountered in patients with DM, especially in those with genetic syndromes of insulin resistance and metabolic syndrome. It is characterised by a velvety, papillomatous, usually pigmented, overgrowth of the epidermis and occurs particularly in the axillae, neck, groin and inframammary areas (Figure 8.58). It may be caused by hyperinsulinaemia-induced stimulation of insulin-like growth factor (IGF)-1 receptors, leading to keratinocyte and dermal fibroblast proliferation.

The skin in diabetes

- Necrobiosis lipoidica diabeticorum
- Diabetic dermopathy
- Diabetic bullae
- Bacterial and *Candida* infection
- Acanthosis nigricans
- Vitiligo
- Eruptive xanthomata
- Necrolytic migratory erythema
- Insulin allergy
- Lipoatrophy
- Lipohypertrophy

Figure 8.57 Many abnormalities of the skin are found in diabetic patients. Some may not be specific to diabetes. Acanthosis nigricans is a skin manifestation of insulin-resistant states, while vitiligo is a cutaneous marker of autoimmunity. Eruptive xanthomata are associated with significant hypertriglyceridaemia. Necrolytic migratory erythema occurs in patients with a glucagonoma and associated diabetes and is very rare. The rashes of insulin allergy, lipoatrophy and lipohypertrophy are all associated with exogenous insulin administration.

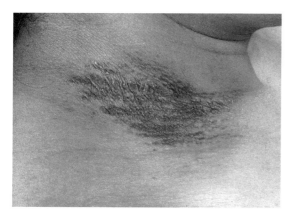

Figure 8.58 Acanthosis nigricans is uncommon. These brown hyperkeratotic plaques with a velvety surface occur most frequently in the axillae and flexures, and on the neck. Acanthosis is associated with insulin resistance caused by genetic defects in the insulin receptor or postreceptor function or the presence of antibodies to the insulin receptor.

Necrobiosis lipoidica diabeticorum

Necrobiosis occurs in 0.3% of diabetic patients with 50% having T1DM. Although traditionally thought of as a classical diabetic skin manifestation, it can also occur in patients without diabetes. Necrobiosis usually develops in young adults or in early middle life and is much more common in women than in men. The skin is the most commonly affected site and the appearance ranges from early dull red papules or plaques to indurated plaques with skin atrophy, often with telangiectatic vessels on a waxy yellowish background to actual skin ulceration (Figures 8.59 and 8.60). Treatment

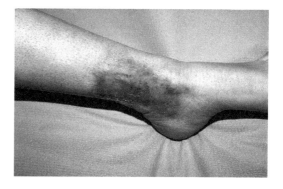

Figure 8.59 A typical lesion of necrobiosis lipoidica diabeticorum on the shin. These lesions are usually non-scaling plaques with yellow atrophic centres and an erythematous edge, and predominantly affect diabetic women. They vary considerably in size, and are often multiple and bilateral. Necrobiosis may occur in non-diabetic subjects.

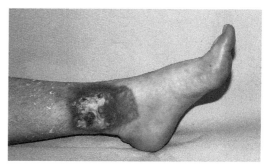

Figure 8.60 Necrobiosis may become severe and ulcerative, causing great distress in affected patients. Spontaneous regression may occur and treatment tends to be unsatisfactory. Skin grafts may become complicated by recurrence within the graft or at an adjacent site.

is controversial, largely unproven and usually ineffective. Intralesional or topical corticosteroids, photochemotherapy or excision and skin grafting may have limited roles.

Diabetic dermopathy

These well-circumscribed, atrophic, brownish scars commonly seen on the shin ('shin spots') occur in up to 50% of diabetic patients (Figure 8.61) and are also seen much less frequently in non-diabetic subjects. Although there is no effective treatment, they tend to regress over time.

Diabetic bullae

Tense blisters, more common in men than women, occurring most frequently on the lower legs and feet, occur rarely in diabetic patients (Figure 8.62). They appear rapidly and heal after a few weeks.

Other

Other skin conditions encountered in diabetic patients are diabetic erythema, periungual telangiectasia, diabetic thick skin (linked with the formation of advanced glycation end-products), vitiligo (autoimmune destruction of melanocytes, Figure 8.63), eruptive xanthomata (caused by hypertriglyceridaemia in diabetic dyslipidaemia,

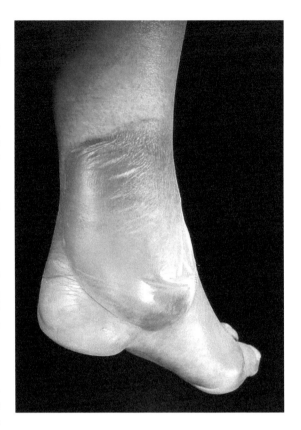

Figure 8.62 Bullous lesions rarely occur in diabetes, and can only be diagnosed when other bullous disorders have been excluded. They usually occur suddenly with no obvious history of trauma and may take a long time to heal. The lower legs and feet are usually affected, and there is a male preponderance.

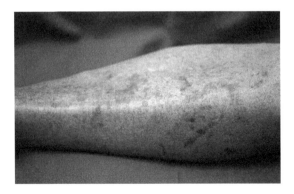

Figure 8.61 Diabetic dermopathy. These pigmented pretibial patches are often seen in diabetic patients, but are not pathognomonic of the disease. There is a male preponderance and the lesions are discrete, atrophic, scaly or hyper-pigmented. The underlying cause is not known.

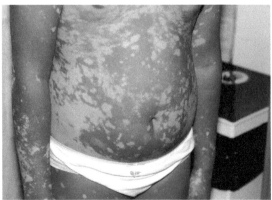

Figure 8.63 Vitiligo, autoimmune destruction of melanocytes, is commonly seen in patients with type 1 diabetes mellitus, itself an autoimmune condition.

Figures 8.64 and 8.65), migratory necrolytic erythema (associated with glucagonoma syndrome, Figure 8.66) and urticarial reactions to insulin allergy. Granuloma annulare (Figure 8.67) has been linked with diabetes but evidence is lacking to prove a true association.

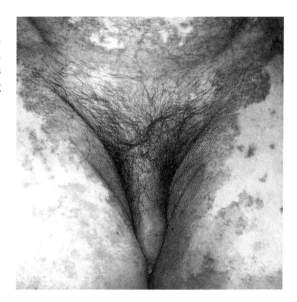

Figure 8.66 Migratory necrolytic erythema. This rash is associated with glucagon-secreting pancreatic tumours (or occasionally zinc deficiency). Such rashes tend to wax and wane in cycles of 1–2 weeks. Diabetes is presumed to be due to increased glucagon-stimulated hepatic gluconeogenesis. Weight loss, diarrhoea and mood changes are frequent features, but death is usually due to massive venous thrombosis. Treatment is by zinc supplementation, or somatostatin or a somatostatin analogue.

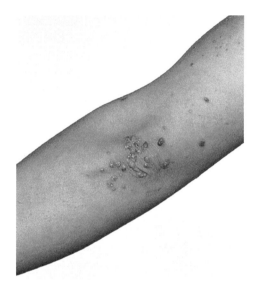

Figure 8.64 Eruptive xanthomata. Type V hyperlipoproteinaemia with an increase in very-low-density lipoproteins and chylomicrons is often associated with glucose intolerance. This lipoprotein abnormality is accentuated by obesity and alcohol consumption, and may lead to acute pancreatitis and peripheral neuropathy.

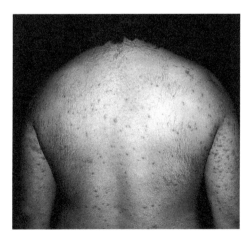

Figure 8.65 Massive eruptive xanthomata in a young man with type 2 diabetes mellitus.

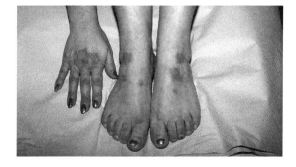

Figure 8.67 Granuloma annulare. Although this skin condition is occasionally seen in diabetic patients, several large studies failed to reveal a significant association between the two disorders, both of which are relatively common.

RARER MANIFESTATIONS OF DIABETES MELLITUS

Diabetic cheiroarthropathy

This rheumatic complication of diabetes manifests itself as limited joint mobility associated with thickening and tightening of the skin, especially noticed on the dorsal surfaces of the hands. Resultant contraction prevents the affected patient from placing their hand flat on to a surface and from approximating the palmar surfaces of the hand—the 'prayer' hand sign (Figure 8.68).

Although seen in both adult-onset T1DM and T2DM, it is most commonly encountered in children and young adults with T1DM, often related to poor glycaemic control and associated with other more specific diabetic complications, such as retinopathy.

Dupuytren's contracture

Dupuytren's contracture (Figure 8.69) has a quoted prevalence varying between 20% and 63% in DM. Furthermore, in patients presenting with Dupuytren's contracture, a high prevalence of diabetes is found. It is more commonly found in elderly patients with a long duration of diabetes and may have an association with carpal tunnel syndrome.

Adhesive capsulitis of the shoulder

There are numerous reports of an association between periarthritis of the shoulder—'frozen shoulder'—and DM, and such patients are encountered frequently in routine diabetic follow-up clinics. This condition is characterised by pain and the limitation of movement of the shoulder joint, both active and passive. Referral to a rheumatologist is appropriate (Figures 8.70–8.73).

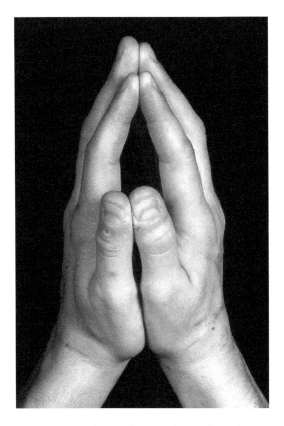

Figure 8.68 Diabetic cheiroarthropathy or limited joint mobility is characterised by an inability to extend fully the metacarpophalangeal and proximal interphalangeal joints when the tips of the fingers and palms of the hands are opposed in the so-called prayer sign. Although it may be seen in adult-onset type 1 and 2 diabetes mellitus, it is most commonly seen in children and young adults with type 1 diabetes mellitus. The development of this abnormality is linked to the duration of diabetes. When present, other diabetic complications are likely to coexist.

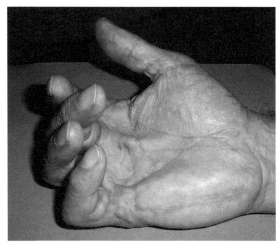

Figure 8.69 Dupuytren's contracture is common in patients with diabetes mellitus. Conversely, in patients presenting with Dupuytren's contracture, a high prevalence of diabetes is found. The exact nature of the link between the two conditions remains unclear.

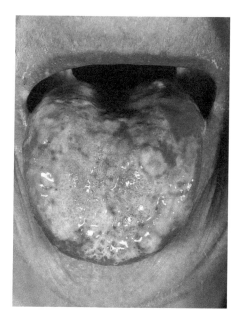

Figure 8.70 Candidiasis is a common fungal infection in diabetic patients. Although particularly common in the vagina or perineum (pruritus vulvae), under the breasts (intertrigo) and on the tip of the penis (balanitis), it may occur elsewhere. The yeasts thrive in glucose-containing media and, hence, control of blood-glucose levels helps to eradicate this troublesome infection. Antifungal creams may be necessary until glucose levels are controlled, but oral antifungal agents are rarely required.

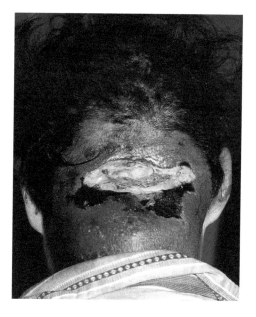

Figure 8.72 Severe bacterial infection in a poorly controlled diabetic patient. Although it is widely believed that diabetic patients are more prone to infection than non-diabetic subjects, it is unclear whether diabetic patients have an increase in the rate of infection in general. Diabetic patients are susceptible to certain infections, including tuberculosis, urinary tract infections and infections due to unusual micro-organisms, such as osteomyelitis, mucormycosis and enterococcal meningitis. Diabetes is thought to impair several aspects of cellular function necessary to combat infection.

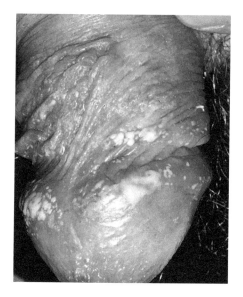

Figure 8.71 Balanitis secondary to diabetes mellitus is a candidal infection of the distal end of the penis and is common at the time of presentation of diabetes in men.

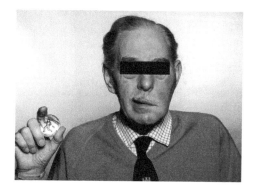

Figure 8.73 Malignant otitis externa. This infection, which can be extremely serious, is almost always due to the *Pseudomonas* species, as was the case here. Affected patients usually have poorly controlled diabetes. This elderly diabetic patient has a seventh cranial nerve palsy as a complication. Antipseudomonal antibiotics and an early surgical opinion are advised.

BIBLIOGRAPHY

Aiello LP, Gardner TW, King GL, et al. Diabetic retinopathy. Diabetes Care. 1998; 21: 143–56

Alexiadou K, Doupis J. Management of diabetic foot ulcers. Diabetes Ther. 2012 Dec: 3(1): 4. Doi: 10.1007/s13300-012-0004-9

Angulo P. Nonalcoholic fatty liver disease. N Engl J Med. 2002; 346: 1221–31

Archer AG, Watkins PJ, Thomas PK, Sharma AK, Payan J. The natural history of acute painful diabetic neuropathy. J Neurol Neurosurg Psychiatr. 1983; 46: 491–9

Arkkila PE, Kantola IM, Viikari JS, et al. Dupuytren's disease in type 1 diabetic patients: A five-year prospective study. Clin Exp Rheumatol. 1996; 14: 59–65

Barnett AH, Dodson PM. Hypertension and Diabetes. London: Science Press Ltd, 1990

Bell DS. Diabetic cardiomyopathy. A unique entity or complication of coronary artery disease? Diabetes Care. 1995; 18: 708–14

British Multicentre Study Group. Photocoagulation for - proliferative diabetic retinopathy: A randomised controlled clinical trial using the zenon arc. Diabetologia. 1984; 26: 109–15

Chauhan A, Foote J, Petch MC, Schofield PM. Hyperinsulinemia, coronary artery disease and syndrome X. J Am Coll Cardiol. 1994; 23: 364–8

Dyck PJ, Thomas PK, Asbury AK, et al. Diabetic Neuropathy. Philadelphia: WB Saunders, 1987

Early Treatment of Diabetic Retinopathy Study Research Group. Photocoagulation for diabetic macular oedema. Arch Ophthalmol. 1985; 103: 1796–806

Edmonds ME. The diabetic foot: Pathophysiology and treatment. Clin Endocrinol Metab. 1993; 15: 889–916

Estacio RO, Schrier RW. Diabetic nephropathy: Pathogenesis, diagnosis, and prevention of progression. Adv Intern Med. 2001; 46: 359–408

Everett E, Mathioudakis N. Update on management of diabetic foot ulcers. Ann NY Acad Sci. 2018 Jan; 1411(1): 153–65. Doi: 10.1111/nyas.13569

Ewing DJ, Campbell IW, Clarke BF. The natural history of diabetic autonomic neuropathy. Q J Med. 1980; 193: 95–108

Finne P, Reunanen A, Stenman S, et al. Incidence of endstage renal disease in patients with Type 1 diabetes. JAMA. 2005; 294: 1782–7

Gross JL, et al. Diabetic nephropathy: Diagnosis, prevention, and treatment. Diabetes Care. 2005 Jan; 28(1): 164–76. Doi: 10.2337/diacare.28.1.164

Ho T, Smiddy WE, Flynn HW Jr. Vitrectomy in the management of diabetic eye disease. Surv Ophthalmol. 1993; 37: 190–202

Javed S, et al. Treatment of painful diabetic neuropathy. Ther Adv Chronic |Dis. 2015 Jan 6(1): 15–28. Doi: 10.1177/2040622314552071

Jelinek JE. The skin in diabetes. Diabetic Med. 1993; 10: 210–13

Jonas JB. Intravitreal triamcinolone acetonide for diabetic retinopathy. Dev Ophthalm. 2007; 39: 96–110. Doi: 10.1159/000098502

Lewis EJ, Hunsicker LG, Pain RP, Rohde RD. The effect of angiotensin-converting enzyme inhibition on diabetic nephropathy. N Engl J Med. 1993; 329: 1456–65

Maiorino MI, et al. Diabetes and sexual dysfunction: Current perspectives. Diabetes Metab Syndr Obes. 2014; 7: 95–105. Doi: 10.2147/DMSO.S36455

Malmberg K. Prospective randomised study of intensive insulin treatment on long term survival after acute myocardial infarction in patients with diabetes mellitus. GIGAMI (Diabetes Mellitus, Insulin Glucose Infusion in Acute Myocardial Infarction) Study Group. Br Med J. 1997; 314: 1512–15

McCulloch DK, Young RJ, Prescott RJ, Clarke BF. The natural history of impotence in diabetic men. Diabetologia. 1984; 26: 437–40

Mogensen CE. Microalbuminuria predicts clinical proteinuria and early mortality in maturity-onset diabetes. N Engl J Med. 1984; 310: 356–60

Mogensen CE, Cooper ME. Diabetic renal disease: From recent studies to improved clinical practice. Diabet Med. 2004; 21: 4–17

Passadakis P, Oreopoulos D. Peritoneal dialysis in diabetic patients. Adv Ren Replace Ther. 2001; 8: 22–41

Passarella P, et al. Hypertension management in diabetes. Diabetes Spectr. 2018 Aug; 31(3): 218–24. Doi: 10.2337/ds17-0085

Perez MI, Kohn SR. Cutaneous manifestations of diabetes mellitus. J Am Acad Dermatol. 1994; 30: 519–31

Reaven GM. Role of insulin resistance in human disease. Diabetes. 1988; 37: 1595–607

Scobie IN, MacCuish AC, Barrie T, et al. Serious retinopathy in a diabetic clinic: Prevalence and therapeutic implications. Lancet. 1981; 2: 520–1

Selby NM, Taal MW. An updated overview of diabetic nephropathy: Diagnosis, prognosis, treatment goals and latest guidelines. Diabetes Obes Metab. 2020, April; 22(Suppl 1): 3–15. Doi: 10.1111/dom.14007

Shapiro LM. A prospective study of heart disease in diabetes mellitus. Q J Med. 1984; 209: 55–68

Solomon SD, Chew E, Duh EJ, Sobrin L, Sun JK, VanderBeek BL, Wykoff CC, Gardner TW. Diabetic retinopathy: A position statement by the American diabetes association. Diabetes Care. 2017; 40(3): 412–18. Doi: 10.2337/dc16-2641

Spruce MC, Potter J, Coppini DV. The pathogenesis of painful diabetic neuropathy: A review. Diabet Med. 2003; 20: 88–98

Stern M. Natural history of macrovascular disease in type 2 diabetes. Role of insulin resistance. Diabetes Care. 1999; 22(Suppl 3): c2–5

Taylor KG, ed. Diabetes and the Heart. Tunbridge Wells: Castle House Publications, 1987

Tomah S, et al. Nonalcoholic fatty liver disease and type 2 diabetes: Where do diabetologists stand. Clin Diabetes Endocrinol 6, 9 (2020). Doi: 10.1186/s40842-020-00097-1

UK Prospective Diabetes Study Group. Efficacy of atenolol and captopril in reducing risk of macrovascular and microvascular complications in type 2 diabetes; UKPDS 39. Br Med J. 1998; 317: 713–20

UK Prospective Diabetes Study Group. Tight blood pressure control and risk of macrovascular and microvascular complications in type 2 diabetes: UKPDS 38. Br Med J. 1998; 317: 703–13

Vinik A, Park TS, Stansberry KB, Pittenger GL. Diabetic neuropathies. Diabetologia. 2000; 43: 957–73

Watkins PJ. The diabetic foot. Br Med J. 2003; 326: 977–9

Young MJ, Boulton AJM, MacLeod AF, et al. A multicentre study of the prevalence of diabetic peripheral neuropathy in the United Kingdom hospital clinic population. Diabetologia. 1993; 35: 150–4

Yusuf S, Sleight P, Pogue J, et al. Effects of an angiotensinconverting-enzyme inhibitor, ramipril, on cardiovascular events in high-risk patients. The heart outcomes prevention evaluation study investigators. N Engl J Med. 2000; 342: 145–53

9

Diabetic dyslipidaemia

Lipid disorders assume a position of utmost importance in patients with diabetes because of the high risk of macrovascular disease in this condition which accounts for 50–70% of deaths. Patients with well-controlled type 1 diabetes mellitus (T1DM) have lipoprotein concentrations similar to the background non-diabetic population. With poor control, increased concentrations of triglyceride-rich lipoproteins are seen, giving rise to hypertriglyceridaemia. However, it is estimated that 30–60% of patients with type 2 diabetes mellitus (T2DM) have hyperlipidaemia. The most common lipoprotein abnormalities in T2DM are increased levels of triglycerides, very-low-density lipoprotein (VLDL) and intermediate-density lipoprotein (IDL) caused by an overproduction of VLDL triglyceride. Low-density lipoprotein (LDL) levels are no different from normal subjects, but a number of potentially atherogenic changes in LDL composition have been observed, particularly a predominance of small dense LDL particles which are known to be particularly atherogenic. The increase in LDL particles, together with the increased VLDL and IDL, leads to an increase in apolipoprotein B levels. The finding of decreased high-density lipoprotein (HDL) concentrations is very prevalent in T2DM, contributing to the atherogenic lipid profile of this disorder. Elevation of postprandial lipids including triglycerides further increases the risk of cardiovascular disease (CVD). The lipid changes of T2DM described previously mimic the lipid changes in obesity and the metabolic syndrome, features frequently seen in patients with T2DM. No consistent change in lipoprotein A (Lp(a)) concentrations has been found in T2DM.

Studies have shown that patients with T2DM benefit at least as much as non-diabetic subjects from lipid-lowering therapy with statins (hydroxy-methylglutaryl-coenzyme A [HMG-CoA] reductase inhibitors). Such agents include simvastatin (Zocor, FloLipid), atorvastatin (Lipitor), pravastatin (Pravachol), pitavastatin (Livalo) and rosuvastatin (Crestor, Ezallor). Simvastatin-treated patients with diabetes in the Scandinavian Simvastatin Survival Study (4S Trial) exhibited reductions in major coronary events and revascularisation procedures of 42% and 48%, respectively. The Collaborative Atorvastatin Diabetes Study (CARDS) included 2838 patients with T2DM and no documented previous history of CVD with at least one of the following features: retinopathy, albuminuria, current smoking or hypertension. Patients had an LDL cholesterol concentration of 4.14 mmol/l (160 mg/dl) or lower. As compared to a placebo, the addition of atorvastatin 10 mg daily led to a 37% reduction in major cardiovascular events and reduced the risk of stroke by 48% with, overall, a highly statistically significant reduction in the composite primary endpoint of acute coronary events, coronary revascularisation and stroke. A 27% decrease in all-cause mortality was also observed, however, this just failed to reach statistical significance. The Cholesterol Treatment Trialists analysed data from 18,686 subjects with diabetes (mostly T2DM) from 14 randomised trials and observed a 9% decrease in all-cause mortality, a 13% decrease in vascular mortality and a 21% decrease in major vascular events per 39 mg/dl (1.01 mmol/l) in LDL cholesterol in the statin-treated group. Similar results were seen in the Heart Protection Study (HPS) in the subgroup with T2DM, with the suggestion that patients with T1DM in the study benefited to the same degree as those with T2DM. Secondary prevention trials

DOI: 10.1201/9781003342700-9

yielded similar results. The results of trials using fibrates as lipid-lowering monotherapy in diabetes have not shown results as robust as the statin trials. In the Fenofibrate Intervention and Event Lowering in Diabetes (FIELD) trial of fenofibrate in 9795 patients between the ages of 50 and 75 with T2DM, there was a reduction of 11% in the primary outcome of coronary events (coronary heart disease death and non-fatal MI (myocardial infarction)) that did not reach statistical significance, although there was a statistically significant decrease in non-fatal MI and total cardiovascular events. A greater reduction in cardiovascular events in patients with high triglyceride levels was noted in the fibrate trials. No useful recent trials of niacin, ezetimibe and PCSK9 inhibitors in diabetic subjects have been reported. No useful benefit of a statin-fibrate combination was demonstrated beyond statin therapy alone. As patients with T2DM are known to be at the same risk of a CVD event as non-diabetic patients with existing CVD, and given the evidence stated here, lipid-lowering therapy is likely to be as clinically effective and cost-effective in patients with T2DM who have not yet sustained a cardiovascular event as in non-diabetic subjects with documented CVD.

The American Diabetes Association (ADA) recommends that all adult patients with diabetes should have a fasting lipid profile at diagnosis to assess their lipid status, repeated every 5 years or sooner as clinically indicated. If statin therapy is instituted, a further profile should be carried out 4–12 weeks after the initiation of treatment. Lifestyle modification focusing on the reduction of saturated fat and cholesterol intake, weight loss (where indicated) and increased physical activity is recommended for diabetic patients with hyperlipidaemia and has been shown to improve the lipid profile. Patients under 40 years of age with cardiovascular risk factors and almost all patients over 40 will end up on statin therapy to prevent CVD. The addition of ezetimibe or a PCSK9 inhibitor should be considered in patients with high cardiovascular risk or very high LDL levels. The American College of Cardiology and The American Heart Association guidelines are similar to the ADA guidelines with a cut-off of a LDL cholesterol of ≥70 mg/dl (1.8 mmol/L), leading to the initiation of statin therapy. A target reduction of LDL cholesterol of 30–49% is recommended, while the ADA recommends a reduction of LDL of 50% in those patients with a 10-year cardiovascular risk >20%.

BIBLIOGRAPHY

Colhoun HM, Betteridge DJ, Durrington PN, et al. Primary prevention of cardiovascular disease with Atorvastatin in Type 2 Diabetes in the Collaborative Atorvastatin Diabetes Study (CARDS): Multicentre randomised placebo-controlled trial. Lancet. 2004; 36: 685–96

Durrington P. Statins and fibrates in the management of diabetic dyslipidemia. Diabet Med. 1997; 14: 513–16

Goldberg RB, Mellies MJ, Sacks FM, et al. Cardiovascular events and their reduction with pravastatin in diabetic and glucose-intolerant myocardial infarction survivors with average cholesterol levels. Circulation. 1998; 98: 2513–19

Haffner SM, Alexander CM, Cook TJ, et al. Reduced coronary events in simvastatin-treated patients with coronary heart disease and diabetes or impaired fasting glucose levels: Sub-group analyses in the Scandinavian Simvastatin Survival Study. Arch Intern Med. 1999; 159: 2661–7

Jialal I, Singh G. Management of diabetic dyslipidemia: An update. World J Diabetes. 2019 May 15; 10(5): 280–90. Doi: 10.4239/wjd.v10.i5.280

Rubins HB, Robins SJ, Collins D, Veterans Affairs High-Density Lipoprotein Cholesterol Intervention Trial Study Group, et al. Gemfibrozil for the secondary prevention of coronary heart disease in men with low levels of high-density lipoprotein cholesterol. N Engl J Med. 1999; 341: 410–18

Steiner G. Lipid intervention trials in diabetes. Diabetes Care. 2000; 23(Suppl 2): B49–53

10

Diabetes and pregnancy

Over the past two decades, there has been a progressive increase in the incidence of both established and gestational diabetes such that almost 1 in 10 pregnancies over the age of 30 are affected by diabetes. The most striking change has been the emergence of type 2 diabetes mellitus (T2DM) in pregnancy as a major clinical issue, reflecting the earlier age of onset of T2DM across the Western world. Of note, in data from the UK National Pregnancy in Diabetes Audit, the median age of women with T2DM in pregnancy was only 34 years, and this group included a higher-than-expected proportion of women from socially deprived backgrounds, reflecting the impact of socioeconomic factors on the development of early type 2 diabetes.

Poor glycaemic control can have an impact on fetal development from the time of conception onwards. The exact mechanisms by which hyperglycaemia impacts fetal development remain poorly understood and may vary across the course of the pregnancy. Thus, in the early weeks after conception, the primary impact may relate direct osmotic effects of glucose and osmotic and oxidative stress associated with hyperglycaemia. Later in pregnancy, following the development of the fetal islets, hyperinsulinaemia may be an important contributor to abnormal fetal growth.

Despite increased understanding of the impact of diabetes on pregnancy, there remains a significantly higher rate of congenital malformations complicating pregnancies, including pre-existing diabetes. The most common anomalies are those affecting the cardiovascular system and central nervous system including ventricular septal defect, patent ductus arteriosus and transposition of the great arteries. Anencephaly and spina bifida are common, with rates reported at greater than 10 times that in the background population in various studies. Given that these abnormalities reflect very early fetal development, optimising blood glucose and diabetes control prior to pregnancy is essential and, similarly, in the preconception period, it is important to consider other risk factors related to pregnancy, including the use of antihypertensive and lipid-lowering medications, which should be stopped prior to conception. There is strong evidence that supplementation with folic acid reduces the risk of neural tube defects and initiation of this prior to conception is now standard practice with the higher dose of 5 mg being recommended.

A specific complication of diabetic pregnancy is the development of macrosomia, defined as a birth weight greater than the 90th percentile of the background population. This can occur in both gestational diabetes and in the context of pregnancy in women with established type 1 and type 2 diabetes present prior to conception. Infants with macrosomia are more likely to have perinatal problems, particularly hypoglycaemia, but also respiratory distress, hyperbilirubinaemia and birth injuries, particularly shoulder dystocia related to increased size at birth. Despite improvements in medical care, macrosomia rates remain very high, with 57% of type 1 and 24% of type 2 pregnancies resulting in a baby who was large for gestational age in a 2020 UK national audit.

There is an increased incidence of early pregnancy loss in diabetes and of preterm labour. At term, there are increased rates of fetal distress with characteristic patterns of recurrent heart decelerations on intrapartum fetal cardiac monitoring, indicating hypoxia. This may reflect a decline in placental function and is particularly seen in the presence of macrosomia. A specific early warning

DOI: 10.1201/9781003342700-10

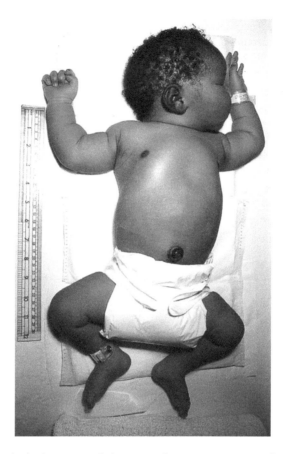

Figure 10.1 A macrosomic baby born to a diabetic mother. Macrosomia reflects suboptimal diabetes control, particularly in late pregnancy, and increased fetal insulin secretion in relation to an increased substrate load. Macrosomia can occur in all types of diabetic pregnancy. Despite advances in diabetes care, it remains common, with some 57% of pregnancies in type 1 mothers resulting in babies who were large for gestational age.

sign of poor placental function in late diabetic pregnancy is a drop in insulin requirements or increased frequency of hypoglycaemia and both should warrant further assessment of fetal health by cardiotocography accompanied by placental ultrasound imaging, where appropriate (Figure 10.1).

MANAGEMENT OF DIABETES IN PREGNANCY

The management of diabetes in pregnancy is aimed at achieving very tight blood-glucose control throughout with target glucose levels of <5.3 mmol/l fasting, <7.8 mmol/l at 1-hour postmeal and <6.4 mmol/l at 2 hours postmeal. These targets are consistent regardless of the type of diabetes. Achieving these targets without problematic

hypoglycaemia can be challenging and is dependent on frequent monitoring. In view of this, the use of continuous glucose-monitoring (CGM) systems has become widespread and, in the UK, is now recommended for the management of women with type 1 diabetes mellitus (T1DM) during pregnancy. This recommendation was based on strong evidence from a UK randomised controlled trial and a Swedish observational study that showed that the use of CGM was associated with greater achievement of glycaemic targets, but also fewer Caesarean sections and neonatal intensive care admissions. For women using CGM, an additional target of achieving more than 70% of time in a target range of 3.5–7.8 mmol/l is also widely advocated.

Diabetes management is based primarily on the use of basal bolus insulin regimes with adjustment of mealtime insulin for carbohydrate. Insulin requirements increase progressively through pregnancy and moderating mealtime carbohydrate portions may be necessary to enable adequate postprandial glucose control. The use of insulin pump and automated insulin-delivery systems in pregnancy is growing and is widely advocated for the management of type 1 patients with problematic hypoglycaemia, which can be a major issue with rapid tightening of blood glucose control. At present, there is limited specific evidence on the role of insulin pump and automated insulin delivery compared to basal bolus insulin regimes on pregnancy outcomes, but several randomised clinical trials of closed-loop technology in pregnancy are in progress.

GESTATIONAL DIABETES

Gestational diabetes mellitus (GDM) is defined as glucose intolerance first appearing in pregnancy and reflects the increased metabolic demands placed on the mother. Following delivery, glucose metabolism returns to normal, but affected women have an increased lifelong risk of subsequent diabetes, with an approximately ten-fold increased risk of diabetes compared to the general population. In some cases, apparent GDM can be the first presentation of T2DM and even T1DM unmasked by the changes occurring in pregnancy. There is now consensus that the diagnosis of gestational diabetes should be based on the results of a 75 g glucose tolerance test with the diagnostic thresholds being a fasting glucose of 5.6 mmol/l or a 2-hour postglucose result of 7.8 mmol/l. UK NICE guidance recommends screening of any women with risk factors for gestational diabetes (including BMI >30, family history of diabetes, ethnicity and a history of macrosomia following a previous pregnancy) at 24–26 weeks' gestation.

Following diagnosis, treatment is based on achieving and sustaining the same glucose controls as used for established diabetes. For many women, this can be achieved with dietary management and the use of metformin which is now accepted as being safe during pregnancy and is widely used. A minority of women (15–30%) require insulin treatment, particularly to optimise postprandial insulin levels and, in some cases, insulin requirements can be very high, reflecting the underlying insulin resistance that underlies gestational diabetes. Without adequate treatment, gestational diabetes carries a similar risk of late pregnancy complications to that seen in established diabetes, with significant rates of adverse outcomes being seen in a meta-analysis of published studies.

BIBLIOGRAPHY

Murphy HR, Howgate C, O'Keefe J et al. Characteristics and outcomes of pregnant women with type 1 or type 2 diabetes: A 5-year national population-based cohort study. Lancet Diabetes Endocrinol. 2021 Mar; 9(3): 153–64. doi: 10.1016/S2213-8587(20)30406-X

NHS Digital 2021. National Pregnancy in Diabetes (NPID) Audit Report 2020. Published Online 14/1021 at https://www.hqip.org.uk/wp-content/uploads/2021/10/REF232_NPID-2020-Report_v20211010_FINAL.pdf

Ye W, Luo C, Huang J, et al. Gestational diabetes mellitus and adverse pregnancy outcomes: Systematic review and meta-analysis. BMJ. 2022; 377. doi: 10.1136/bmj-2021-067946

11

Living with diabetes

In common with other chronic medical conditions, diabetes mellitus impacts on quality of life, sometimes significantly so. The fear of hypoglycaemia (for those patients treated with sulphonylureas or insulin) and concern about glycaemic control and diabetic complications are ever present. Advances in therapeutic agents, such as novel insulin preparations, have undoubtedly improved diabetic patients lives, while the advent of insulin pen devices to administer insulin was a great step forward for insulin-treated patients followed by insulin-pump therapy. Perhaps the greatest revolution in the care of people with diabetes has been the relatively recent introduction of sturdy and reliable systems of relatively non-invasive continuous glucose monitoring. Complications of diabetes such as visual impairment due to retinopathy, neuropathy, nephropathy and erectile dysfunction clearly have a significant effect on the quality of diabetic patients' lives. The diagnosis of diabetes invokes stress in affected individuals. In one study, at the time of diagnosis of type 1 diabetes mellitus (T1DM), 36% of children exhibited significant psychological distress. Remarkably, however, in 93%, this had completely abated 9 months after diagnosis. Not surprisingly, the parents of newly diagnosed children also experience psychological upset of a temporary nature, more prominent in mothers. Adults with new-onset T1DM have similar temporary psychological responses. The diagnosis of gestational diabetes mellitus is associated with increased maternal anxiety and stress. It has been suggested that stressful experiences may lead to an increased risk of developing both T1DM and type 2 diabetes mellitus (T2DM).

The prevalence of depression is two to three times higher in people with diabetes compared to the non-diabetic population, with many cases going unrecognised. Meta-analyses have suggested that the global prevalence of depression in people with T2DM has increased from 20% in 2007 to 32% in 2018. A recent study showed that people who develop T2DM at an age less than 40 years have a greater risk of developing depression than those diagnosed at 50 years or greater. Interestingly, depression commonly precedes the diagnosis in T2DM patients, as previously mentioned. The course of depression in diabetes may be particularly chronic, and severe and depression is associated with adverse glycaemic control and clinical outcomes. Separate from depression, studies have identified a high prevalence of diabetes distress, defined as patient concerns about disease management, support, emotional burden and access to care, affecting one in four patients with T1DM and one in five with T2DM. Such patients may be identified using simple scales in clinical practice (Diabetes Distress Scale, Problem Areas in Diabetes [PAID] Scale). The diagnosis of diabetes affects other aspects of the diabetic patient's life. In most developed countries, drivers with diabetes have a statutory requirement to declare their diabetes to the national licensing authority. Furthermore, failure to do so may invalidate motor insurance policies. Following declaration of the diagnosis of diabetes, a driving licence is issued for a maximum of 3 years in the UK, but is renewable at no cost following completion of a medical questionnaire. In the UK, if an insulin-treated diabetic patient has one severe hypoglycaemic event, defined as an event requiring third-party assistance, the patient must stop driving and inform the licensing authority (DVLA). If there is more than one severe hypoglycaemic event in any 12-month period, the licence will be revoked and a medical opinion sought. For patients who drive large vehicles, they must stop driving after one such event and inform the DVLA. For such patients, licences are issued on an annual basis. Most countries impose limitations on the issue of vocational licences (heavy goods vehicles, passenger carrying vehicles) to insulin-treated diabetic drivers. In 2012, the UK followed Canada in allowing insulin-treated diabetic patients to fly commercial aircraft as long as there was a second pilot in the cockpit and subject to strict conditions including frequent blood glucose monitoring, which was greatly assisted by the introduction of modern continuous glucose monitoring systems. In the US, the Federal Aviation Administration followed suit in 2019. In a similar vein, such patients are now able to become air traffic controllers. Diabetic patients may experience difficulties with employment. Statutory or company policy make employment in certain occupations, such as off-shore work, difficult. However, progress in this area is being made, particularly in the UK with the advent of the Equality Act 2010, which renders it against the law for an employer to discriminate because of a disability. In many cases, people with diabetes will be covered by the current definition of disability, helping them in potential employment scenarios. Nevertheless, some countries do not allow employment in the armed forces. In the US armed forces, diabetes remains a disqualifying health condition. Furthermore, even when there is no risk due to possible hypoglycaemia, discrimination by employers may affect hiring practices, leading to loss of self-esteem and earning ability, impacting the patient's ability to support a family and their future quality of life.

Insurance may also pose problems for individuals with diabetes. Diabetic patients may experience difficulty obtaining life insurance on favourable terms. More favourable insurance terms may be provided by approved brokers recommended by national diabetes associations. In the UK, most car insurance companies no longer penalise people with diabetes by charging higher premiums.

There are many other areas in life where having diabetes may cause difficulties, including travel overseas, insurance and medical care abroad, exposure to unusual foods and drinks in different countries and the effect of intercurrent illness and sport on day-to-day blood glucose control.

BIBLIOGRAPHY

Dibato J, et al. Temporal trends in the prevalence and incidence of depression and the interplay of comorbidities in patients with young- and usual-onset type 2 diabetes from the USA and the UK. Diabetologia. 2022; 65: 2066–77. Doi: 10.1007/s00125-022-05764-9

Kovacs M, Goldston D, Obrosky DS, Bonar LK. Psychiatric disorders in youths with IDDM: Rates and risk factors. Diabetes Care. 1997; 20: 36–44

Russell-Jones DL, et al. Pilots flying with insulin-treated diabetes. Diabetes Obes Metab. 2021 Jul; 23(7): 1439–44. Doi: 10.1111/dom.14375

12

Future developments in diabetes care

TOWARDS A CURE FOR TYPE 1 DIABETES MELLITUS: TRANSPLANTATION

Whole-pancreas and islet transplantation are now well established as a management strategy for type 1 diabetes mellitus (T1DM). Whole-pancreas transplantation was first performed in 1964 and since then more than 60,000 transplants have been performed. The majority of these have been performed as a combined procedure in patients requiring a renal transplant for end-stage diabetic nephropathy, with a minority being conducted for diabetes control alone. Recent data on outcomes are favourable, with 73% insulin independence at 5 years postprocedure for combined kidney and pancreas grafts, with a lower graft survival rate and insulin independence of 53% being reported for pancreas transplant alone. Given that the procedure has a significant mortality and morbidity, its use for the primary management of diabetes in the absence of renal failure has become less widespread with the establishment of islet transplantation.

After several false starts, the modern era of islet transplantation began with refinement of islet isolation techniques in the 1990s and the publication of the first consistently successful series of islet transplants by a group led by James Shapiro from Edmonton, Canada, in 2000. In contrast to earlier attempts, the transplantation was based on a steroid-free immunosuppression regime, resulting in a lower metabolic demand on the transplanted islets associated with corticosteroid treatment. In the initial publication from this group, seven consecutive transplanted patients achieved insulin independence after one or two infusions of donor islets and, following this early success, the 'Edmonton protocol' was widely adopted in transplant centres across the world with more than 1000 recipients being included in an international registry of islet transplantation.

Islet cells are obtained from a donated human pancreas by a process of partial pancreatic digestion and a differential centrifugation. The isolated and purified islets are then administered into the hepatic portal system when grafting takes place. Successful islet transplantation is associated with insulin independence, but there remain limitations to the technique. To obtain an adequate islet mass to achieve insulin dependence, most recipients require at least two separate islet donations and the supply of human islets remains scarce (Figures 12.1 and 12.2).

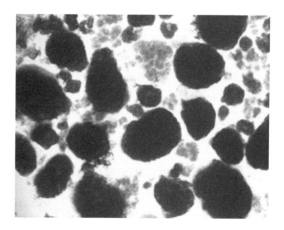

Figure 12.1 Isolated human islet cells prepared transplantation. The islets are isolated from a donated human pancreas by a process of partial digestion and ultracentrifugation in a cooled centrifuge. The retrieval of good-quality islets from a donor pancrease is critical to the success of islet cell transplantation.

DOI: 10.1201/9781003342700-12

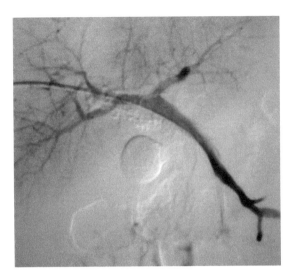

Figure 12.2 A portal venogram showing the hepatic portal vein prior to administration of isolated human islets. In the Edmonton protocol, an adequate mass of freshly isolated islets is infused through a catheter placed into the main portal vein.

Since the initial Edmonton protocol, there have been further refinements in the immunosuppression protocols used for islet transplantation, with more intensive T-cell depletion at the induction of immunosuppression being widely favoured. Overall, results from transplantation are good with about 75% of patients achieving insulin independence in recent series, and with about half of recipients achieving long-term insulin independence. Even among those who do not achieve insulin independence, significant improvements in glycaemic control were achieved and sustained, with long-term freedom from severe hypoglycaemia being achieved in the majority of patients, regardless of whether insulin independence is achieved. The overall duration of insulin independence is variable, with median rates of insulin independence of between 40% and 60% being reported at 3 to 5 years in different cohorts. In contrast, freedom from hypoglycaemia among recipients who have had recurrent severe hypoglycaemia prior to transplantation is sustained beyond 5 years in the majority of recipients.

There remain significant limitations to islet transplantation which mean that it has remained a niche treatment for a small number of people with T1DM. The need for lifelong immunosuppression is associated with significant risks including an increased risk of malignancy, particularly for skin cancers and lymphoma. Furthermore, the available supply of human islets remains small and is likely to remain a limiting factor in the long term.

In view of this, the primary indication for islet transplantation remains for patients with intractable, recurrent severe hypoglycaemia that persists despite optimised medical management including use of insulin-pump and sensor technology. A secondary indication is in the management of patients with suboptimal glucose control who have previously received a kidney transplant and are, thus, already on immunosuppression. Islet after kidney (IAK) transplantation is increasingly being used to optimise diabetes in such patients and carries a more favourable risk–benefit ratio through not requiring additional long-term immunosuppression and through the potential to improve renal graft survival through improved diabetes control.

Presently, the strongest evidence for the benefits of islet transplantation is in the context of the management of hypoglycaemia, with long-term freedom from hypoglycaemia seen in recipients. Ongoing research in this field aims to improve islet survival and duration of insulin independence. This is focused on a greater understanding of the immune response that ultimately leads to islet loss and recurrence of T1DM and also on understanding the impact of additional cellular factors that help support islet cell survival and function.

More widespread use of islet cell therapy will require improvements in immunosuppression, islet graft survival and alternative sources of islets other than cadaveric human donor tissue. While various studies have explored encapsulation of islets and use of humanised porcine islets, the greatest interest, at present, is in the potential for bioengineered human beta cells (β-cells) and differentiated islets derived from embryonic stem-cells. Two companies ViaCell and Vertex have recently performed first-in-man studies and, of particular note, Vertex presented data showing a therapeutic effect in a single patient with a marked reduction in insulin requirements, though not complete insulin independence. Based on these preliminary results, the United States Food and

Drug Administration (FDA) has granted investigational status for a novel device comprising Vertex' encapsulated embryonic stem-cell-derived islets, which is now entering Phase 1/2 clinical trials as a potential treatment for T1DM.

T1DM PREVENTION

Greater understanding of the immune processes underlying the onset of T1DM has now led to the development of the first proven treatment to attenuate the immune response. The drug teplizumab, a humanised anti-CD3 monoclonal antibody, delays overt T1DM in at-risk individuals. It received FDA approval in 2022 after a 10-year development programme and is now starting to enter clinical practice. In clinical trials, teplizumab was associated with delay in the progression of diabetes by more than 2 years, with preservation of some β-cell function as measured by C-peptide production. This gives the potential for using immunotherapy to alter the natural history of T1DM, as existing evidence has shown that preservation of some β-cell function and C-peptide positivity is associated with reduced risk of complications and better overall glycaemic stability with less hypoglycaemia. A future challenge in immunotherapy will be to determine screening strategies for the very early detection of T1DM in the population, as such treatment would be most effective when the earliest changes in glucose metabolism occur and while β-cell mass is well preserved. Another challenge will be to bring down the extreme cost of immunotherapy, which, at present, would limit its uptake.

TYPE 2 DIABETES MELLITUS: SURGICAL AND ENDOSCOPIC INTERVENTIONS

A major area of advancement in type 2 diabetes mellitus (T2DM) has been the recognition of the importance of the gut and gut hormones in the aetiology of insulin resistance and dysglycaemia. Much has been learned from the field of bariatric surgery, which has been shown capable of reversing T2DM independent of its effect on weight. Multiple studies have shown that for patients with

obesity, surgical intervention can be more effective than pharmacotherapy. These observations were initially made in patients with a BMI >35 and have now been extended to those with a BMI in the range of 30–35, which, while still within the diagnostic criteria for obesity, is below the level at which surgical intervention would be considered. Data from observational studies, notably the Swedish Obesity Study, have shown that surgical treatment, particularly in the early years after diabetes, is associated with improved glucose control, reduction in requirement for pharmacotherapy and, in some cases, reversal of T2DM. Furthermore, long-term follow up in the Swedish cohort has shown that early surgery is associated with a reduction in microvascular complications and cardiovascular morbidity. Of note, improvements in blood glucose control and a reduction in insulin requirements are observed very early after surgery and before major weight loss has occurred. This has led to interest in the underlying mechanisms by which bariatric surgery improves glycaemia, and studies in animals and, in some cases in man, have identified multiple changes that may influence glucose homeostasis. Given these extensive effects, it has been suggested that the term 'metabolic' rather than 'bariatric' surgery may be more appropriate to describe surgical management aimed primarily at reversal or management of diabetes (Figure 12.3).

The surgical procedures with the greatest impact on metabolic parameters are those that involve the duodenum and this has led to particular interest in the study of the duodenum's role in glucose metabolism and its identification as a potential target for diabetes interventions. Studies in rodent models showed that a high fat and sucrose diet leads to a thickening of the duodenal mucosa and that this is associated with the development of insulin resistance and associated metabolic derangement. Ablation of the mucosa was shown to reverse these changes and, based on these observations, a therapeutic intervention has been developed. This intervention, Revita Duodenal Mucosal Resurfacing (DMR) is an endoscopic technique by which a balloon catheter is placed in the duodenum and inflated with heated saline to produce a focal thermal injury and ablate the mucosal surface. In initial randomised controlled trials, DMR

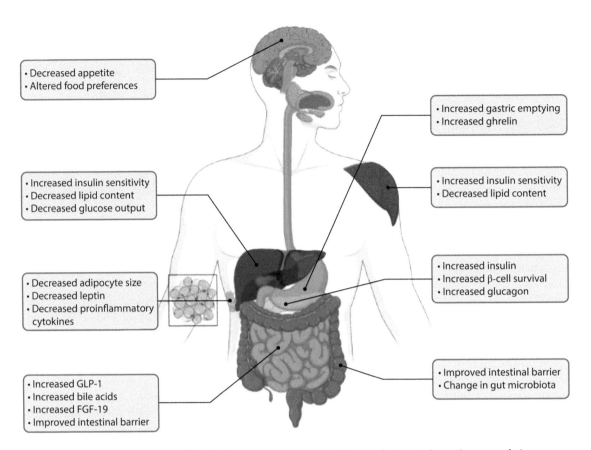

- Decreased appetite
- Altered food preferences

- Increased gastric emptying
- Increased ghrelin

- Increased insulin sensitivity
- Decreased lipid content
- Decreased glucose output

- Increased insulin sensitivity
- Decreased lipid content

- Decreased adipocyte size
- Decreased leptin
- Decreased proinflammatory cytokines

- Increased insulin
- Increased β-cell survival
- Increased glucagon

- Increased GLP-1
- Increased bile acids
- Increased FGF-19
- Improved intestinal barrier

- Improved intestinal barrier
- Change in gut microbiota

Figure 12.3 Putative actions of bariatric surgery on metabolic regulation: A broad range of changes have been described following Roux-en-Y gastric bypass, which may explain the impact of surgery to improve diabetes control.

treatment was associated with improvements in glucose control and insulin resistance. Of particular note, DMR was associated with a reduction in liver fat content and improvements in liver transaminases in patients with elevated baseline liver fat content, suggesting a potential benefit in the management of non-alcoholic fatty liver disease, which is an increasing issue in T2DM. DMR has now entered clinical practice in some regions. Other techniques involving ablation of the duodenal mucosa, including radiofrequency ablation (repurposing a technique developed for treatment of oesophageal dysplasia), are also in development. Another approach to manipulation of the duodenum that has entered clinical practice is the EndoBarrier duodeno-jejunal bypass liner (GI Dynamics, Boston, US), which was developed primarily to support weight loss. The EndoBarrier is a 60 cm-long polymer tube that is placed endoscopically into the duodenum and anchored at the duodenal bulb, allowing nutrients to pass directly from the stomach into the jejunum. This is left in place for up to 1 year and then removed at a further endoscopy. The outcomes associated with the use of the device were variable, with a multicentre trial showing no improvement in glycaemic control over standard treatments, whereas significant improvements in weight and glycemic control were observed and maintained for up to 3 years in a UK clinical practice series of patients with longer-duration diabetes that had proved refractory to standard treatment (Figures 12.4 and 12.5).

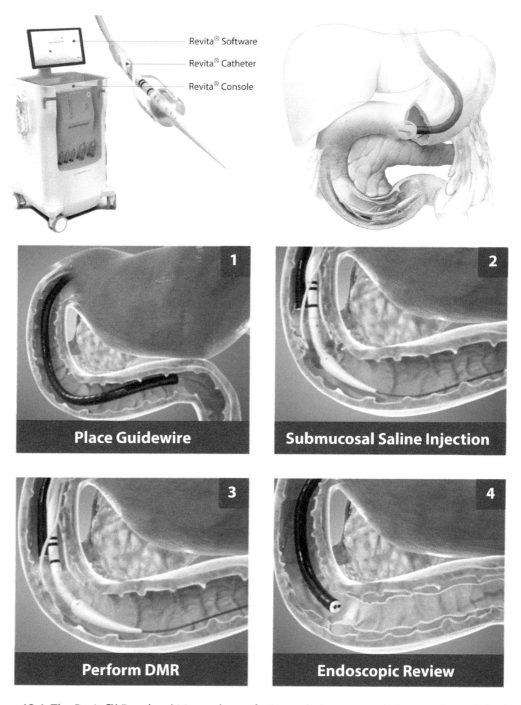

Figure 12.4 The Revita™ Duodenal Mucosal resurfacing technique uses a balloon catheter linked to a computerized operating console (top left) to deliver a thermal injury to the duodenal mucosa. The catheter is placed endoscopically and under x-ray guidance into the duodenum (top right, 1). The mucosa is separated from the underlying submucosa by a local injection of saline (2) and the catheter balloon is inflated with heated saline to produce a focal thermal injury, which leads to atrophy and regrowth of the mucosa (3). The balloon catheter is then removed and the mucosa inspected before withdrawal of the endoscope (4). The resultant 'resurfacing' of the mucosa is associated with changes in multiple metabolic parameters including improved glycaemic control and reduced liver fat.

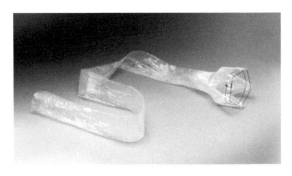

Figure 12.5 The EndoBarrier™ duodeno-jejunal barrier liner is inserted endoscopically into the duodenum, creating a barrier between nutrients passing from the stomach to duodenum which are prevented from reaching the duodenal mucosa.

BIBLIOGRAPHY

Bellin MD, Dunn TB. Transplant strategies for type 1 diabetes: Whole pancreas, islet and porcine beta cell therapies. Diabetologia. 2020; 63: 2049–56. doi: 10.1007/s00125-020-05184-7

Butler PC, Gale EA. Reversing type 1 diabetes with stem cell-derived islets: A step closer to the dream? J Clin Invest. 2022 Feb 1; 132(3): e158305. doi: 10.1172/JCI158305

Carlsson LMS, Sjöholm K, Karlsson C, et al. Long-term incidence of microvascular disease after bariatric surgery or usual care in patients with obesity, stratified by baseline glycaemic status: A post-hoc analysis of participants from the Swedish Obese Subjects study. Lancet Diabetes Endocrinol. 2017 Apr; 5(4): 271–9. doi: 10.1016/S2213-8587(17)30061-X

Cummings DE, Rubino F. Metabolic surgery for the treatment of type 2 diabetes in obese individuals. Diabetologia. 2018 Feb; 61(2): 257–64. doi: 10.1007/s00125-017-4513-y

Hering BJ, Ballou CM, Bellin MD, et al. Factors associated with favourable 5-year outcomes in Islet Transplant alone recipients with type 1 diabetes complicated by severe hypoglycaemia in the Collaborative Islet Transplant Registry. Diabetologia. 2023 Jan;66(1):163–173. doi: 10.1007/s00125-022-05804-4

Mingrone G, van Baar AC, Devière J, et al. Safety and efficacy of hydrothermal duodenal mucosal resurfacing in patients with type 2 diabetes: The randomised, double-blind, sham-controlled, multicentre REVITA-2 feasibility trial. Gut. 2022 Feb; 71(2): 254–64. doi: 10.1136/gutjnl-2020-323608

Ruban A, Miras A, Glaysher MA, et al. Duodenal-jejunal bypass liner for the management of type 2 diabetes mellitus and obesity: A multicenter randomized controlled trial. Annal Surg. 2022 March; 275(3): 440–47. doi: 10.1097/SLA.0000000000004980

Ryder REJ, Yadagiri M, Burbridge W, et al. Duodenal-jejunal bypass liner for the treatment of type 2 diabetes and obesity: 3-year outcomes in the First National Health Service (NHS) EndoBarrier Service. Diabet Med. 2022 Jul; 39(7): e14827. doi: 10.1111/dme.14827

Shapiro AMJ, Lakey JRT, Ryan EA, et al. Islet transplantation in seven patients with type 1 diabetes mellitus using a glucocorticoid-free immunosuppressive regimen. N Engl J Med. 2000; 343: 230–23. doi: 10.1056/NEJM200007273430401

Tatovic D, Dayan CM. Replacing insulin with immunotherapy: Time for a paradigm change in type 1 diabetes. Diabet Med. 2021; 38: e14696. doi:10.1111/dme.14696

van Baar ACG, Meiring S, Holleman F, et al. Alternative treatments for type 2 diabetes and associated metabolic diseases: Medical therapy or endoscopic duodenal mucosal remodelling? Gut. 2021 Nov; 70(11): 2196–204. doi: 10.1136/gutjnl-2020-323931

Index